Dissolve Fat
and Eliminate Cellulite!

Gerald M. Parker, D.O.

Foreword by
Michael Steelman, M.D.

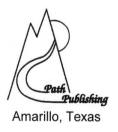

Path Publishing

Amarillo, Texas

Originally printed 2005

Path Publishing, Inc.
4302 W. 51st #121
Amarillo, Texas 79109-6159
USA
www.pathpublishing.com
path2@pathpublishing.com

ISBN 978-1-891774-03-4
ISBN 1-891774-03-4

Printed in the United States of America

10 9 7 6 5 4 3

Contents

Foreword

By Michael Steelman, M.D.

The numbers are staggering and frightening. More than two of every three American adults are overweight or obese. Excess pounds are associated with heart disease, high blood pressure, diabetes, gallbladder problems, back strain, various forms of cancer, and significant psychosocial disability and discomfort. It has been estimated that 400,000 excess deaths per year in our country are due to the effects of obesity, making it the largest cause of death in America.

My interest in weight problems began when, as a young family physician, I noticed many of my patients would be better treated by weight loss than by the various and expensive medications they were taking. Like most physicians, my medical education barely discussed nutritional issues. I only had one lecture on weight problems; it dealt mostly with rare genetic and glandular disorders I have yet to see in more than thirty years of practice.

I found the problems of overweight patients intriguing and began a personal journey to learn everything I could to help them. For the past twenty years, my professional career has been devoted entirely to the problems of the overweight and obese.

This journey recently led me to the doorstep of Dr. Gerald Parker to learn the art and science of Mesotherapy. He personally took the challenge to heart and served as my teacher, coach and mentor. He sees his patients as unique individuals, and approaches them with expert knowledge, a balance of hopeful and realistic expectations, and the warmth of compassion. Those characteristics will reach out to the reader as well.

Such attributes are quite valuable in this field since attempts at weight management are often frustrating for patients and physicians alike. Our society pressures us (especially females) to be sleek and slender while simultaneously foisting upon us a plethora of tasty, but unhealthy, foods. Thanks to the efforts of the nation's farmer, food is abundant and inexpensive. As portion sizes increase, so do our waistlines.

Food is a symbol for love, nurturing, friendship, and more. We eat for a variety of emotional reasons and center our holidays and other celebrations around a communal feast. When someone dies, we take food to the grieving family.

Until recently, the conventional wisdom was that weight problems were merely a character issue, a lack of will power. Medical students were taught that fat cells had no functions except to store fat. Now we know that genetics and individual biochemistry play an important role in weight management and that the fat cell is a hotbed of activity, producing a variety of hormones and other substances that have very important functions in the body.

Much has been learned, but it is still generally accepted that only 5 to 10 percent of overweight people will reach their goal weight and keep it off.

It is particularly frustrating for a person to lose a considerable amount of weight and still have areas of their body with excessive fatty deposits — love handles, tummy rolls, saddlebags, and cellulite. Even in people at a relatively normal weight, these cosmetic flaws can take a toll on self-esteem and lower the quality of life, especially in our appearance-conscious society.

Mesotherapy is particularly valuable as an adjunct in the treatment of such problems. In this book, Dr. Parker deftly navigates a discussion of this procedure much like he navigated his way from the plains of Amarillo, Texas, to the city lights of Paris, France, to learn Mesotherapy from the world's acknowledged leading authority.

Dr. Parker is direct and plainspoken in his discussion about the proper role of Mesotherapy and which people are most likely to benefit. He describes the characteristics to look for in a Mesotherapist and the ways to maximize the results. In these discussions, he is absolutely "on the mark."

With any new procedure (and Mesotherapy is new in the United States, even though its much longer European history is detailed within), patients and physicians alike should ask two questions: Is it effective? Is it safe?

One only needs to read the testimonials in Chapter 15 to find the answer to the first question. Dr. Parker details the results of his own clinical research as well.

Likewise, Dr. Parker clearly addresses the safety issue. He discusses the various compounds used, the follow-up measures needed, *and* the value of finding a physician who understands weight management and who has been properly trained.

Mesotherapy is a technique that bridges the gap between health and appearance. It is a procedure that turns frowns of frustration into smiles of success. It is a tool that lets us put finishing touches on our personal remodeling project.

Mesotherapy is one piece of the puzzle of weight management. Dr. Parker is one of America's preeminent experts in this field and is a pioneer who, in the pages that follow, has placed that piece squarely in its proper place.

Acknowledgements

My greatest thanks go to Dr. Jacque LeCoz. Considered the foremost authority on Mesotherapy in the world, he has been so gracious in letting me train under him in Paris. He has become a friend with whom I have had the pleasure of visiting at various seminars in Canada and the United States.

An excellent teacher, he was very patient with me while he translated everything from French to English. He also arranged for me to spend time with other Mesotherapy physicians in France.

I would also like to thank Dr. Michael Pistor, the forerunner of modern Mesotherapy who gave the science its name, and doctors I spent time with in France: Dr. Philippe Berthier, Dr. Philippe Fabri, and Dr. Florence Thomas.

A special thank-you goes to Dr. Patricia Rittes of Brazil for her kind encouragement, and for her lead worldwide in Meso-Lipotherapy techniques.

Other physicians that deserve special thanks for helping spread the word about Mesotherapy are Dr. Abdula Kalil, Dr. Roman Chubaty, Dr. Juan Carlos Mendez, Dr. Scott Greenberg, Dr. Lionel Bissoon, and Dr. John Taylor, my partner of many years. A better partner I could not find.

Thanks to the American Society of Bariatric Physicians, who invited me to speak at a recent annual meeting where hundreds of physicians were anxious to hear the latest innovations in this exciting therapy.

I am especially grateful to Dr. Michael Steelman, Dr. Denise Bruner, Dr. Larry Richardson, Dr. Gary Albertson,

Dr. Harold Seim and all of the other physicians who joined me for my first physician training session in Dallas, Texas. These physicians and others listed at the end of this book will be very helpful if you ever need someone to give you advice.

THANKS TO FAMILY AND STAFF

I especially thank my wife and children who have been so supportive. My wonderful wife Linda has taken much of my share of the household chores while I have been traveling around the world gathering information and training. She has stood by my side through thick and thin, all the while telling me everything would be OK.

To Kim, my fantastic daughter who convinced me to go to France.

To Sandy, my brilliant daughter who went to France with me on the first trip and helps with all of the physician training seminars.

To my son Zack and his wife Jill who have helped immensely in setting up the training sessions so I can concentrate on the training itself.

To my son Kevin and his wife Christen, both equally extraordinary, who prepare the PowerPoint presentations, invaluable tools for training other physicians at seminars around the country.

To Gary and Josh, my indispensable sons-in-law who help take care of things while I am away from home. Thank you for doing everything with smiles on your faces.

To my awe-inspiring grandchildren with whom God has blessed me. I love them all so much, and I am going to try to spend more time with each one of them in the near future.

Finally, to Robin Malatesta for deciphering my handwriting and listening to my voice on countless hours of audio tapes, turning all of that into something you, dear reader, can actually understand.

Disclaimer

This book is for informational purposes only, to educate people about the procedure called Mesotherapy. If you require diagnosis, treatment, correction of lifestyle, change of diet, exercise guidance, or any other medical advice, you need to see a physician personally.

If you are a physician, please be informed that the procedures discussed in this book should not be done without specific training and understanding of the procedures and medications used. This book is not a substitute for training. It is a patient education tool. You should not consider the material in this book to be a practice of medicine, but only for guidance of patients considering Mesotherapy and wanting more information.

I hope Appendix 1 helps you find a physician practicing Mesotherapy in your area.

And I hope Appendix 2 aids you in a search to obtain supplements mentioned in this book. Although most of them can be obtained without a prescription, I strongly encourage you to work with a physician when you use any of them.

Introduction

As a practicing physician, I have spent a lot of time traveling and learning new techniques from other physicians. Every time I hear or read about something that might help my patients, I set my mind to finding out more about it. This often leads me to a seminar in some other city or state, and a few times to other countries. My goal is to discover what therapies are available for my patients.

I have been blessed with a partner, Dr. John Taylor, who has this same philosophy. It seems that one of us is always disappearing so we can learn about some new technique, therapy, or approach. In the search for the "new" we often find ourselves being presented with something we heard about years earlier. Sometimes we research techniques for years before we jump in. It is all about total reliability and timing.

I have traveled to learn about acupuncture, hyperbaric oxygen, Prolotherapy, allergy testing and treatments, chelation, and numerous other techniques that could be beneficial. For instance, the most advanced training for acupuncture is not here in the United States, and I was fortunate to find leading experts from China, Japan, and Australia giving demonstrations in Vancouver, British Columbia.

I vividly remember the Chinese doctor who knew more about the treatment than the other two but had limited English skills. And I understood not one syllable of Chinese. As it turned out, the Australian doctor, who knew the least of the three, was able to explain everything in terms I could understand.

I was then impressed as I watched the hands-on demonstrations of the Chinese and Japanese doctors, since I could finally understand what they were doing, and nonverbal communication made training possible.

When I first became interested in using a technique for spot fat reduction called Mesotherapy, I was a little distraught to find out that the world's foremost authority on the treatment, Dr. Jacque LeCoz, was a Frenchman who was planning no speaking engagements in North America anytime soon. And, I deduced that he probably spoke very little English. Worry set in. I had flashbacks of the Chinese acupuncture trip. But reason gave way to history and I decided I *must* go to France. France is, after all, where Mesotherapy was born. Safe to say, anyone doing Mesotherapy for any length of time had been doing it in France.

Still, I was a little hesitant. I am not, you see, a world traveler — a few trips to Canada and one mission trip to Mexico with translator in tow so no language mishaps there. But France?

In high school, I took French. Unfortunately, my motive was to gain a credit, not learn a language. Mr. Bentley's French class was comprised mostly of girls who were also in his drama class. So about all I had to do to get a decent grade was help with various play preparations. Every week he would write lessons on the board in both French and English and I would learn them by rote. Home free, because Mr. Bentley rarely gave tests. Whenever he set a test date there was a good chance the girls would sweet-talk him out of it by saying they needed to study their lines for a play. He would capitulate, I could relax, and overall I learned nothing.

Picture a father and daughter coming out of a subway tunnel in the middle of a busy downtown street, four large suitcases in their possession. They have no idea where they are or how to get to where they need to be. They ask for directions, but no one can help them. So they set out on their own, in a huge, strange, crazy city. Look at their faces: pure bewilderment.

Those two people are my daughter and me alone in Paris. I asked Sandy to come with me. I hoped she could learn about Mesotherapy, help me with the language barrier, and figure out where we were and what were we doing there.

No, she had never even had French in high school, but I bought her a French/American dictionary and hoped her keen intelligence would carry us through. You know, those dictionaries are not as helpful as one might think.

But there is such a thing as luck, or good fortune. Even though we were in Paris almost immediately after the start of the war with Iraq, and Americans were not popular in France, on occasion someone could understand us and lead us toward the address we showed them.

To my great amazement and even greater thankfulness, Dr. LeCoz spoke English fairly well. Sometimes he or I would ask, "What's the word for...?" But we managed nicely. LeCoz was very generous with his time, talent and training. Not only did he make himself available to train me, but he also made it possible for me to visit with other physicians in Paris who made Mesotherapy a part of their practices.

Yet my good fortune did not stop there. I was allowed to spend an entire day at the Institute of National Sports Education Physique, the French equivalent of our National Olympic Training Center. All the top French athletes trained there.

When athletes are in the middle of training, they don't want to stop and deal with mild injuries, of course. While most conventional treatments for even minor sports injuries require days or weeks for treatment and recovery, Mesotherapy allows the athlete to continue with training while treating the injury. So it has in a way revolutionized sports injury treatment.

Along the way, I found out there was a physician even more experienced than Dr. LeCoz in the science of spot fat reduction. As soon as I returned to the States, I sought out Dr. Patricia Rittes, a Brazilian doctor who has performed more than 26,000 treatments on body fat and more than 2,000 eye-fat pad treatments. She and other physicians have reported excellent results in the treatment of fat areas just about anywhere on the body — abdomen, spare tires, love handles, inner and outer thighs, double chins, and the pad areas under the eyes. I felt very fortunate to spend time training under Dr. Rittes!

Meanwhile, Dr. LeCoz has become a good friend, and has solicited my help when he gives seminars in the United States. I feel honored that he has enough confidence in my ability to have me demonstrate for him.

CHAPTER I

Different Techniques — Different Results

Through my contacts with Dr. LeCoz, I now know there are many physicians around the world with knowledge of Mesotherapy. And, in general practice, though many variations in the medications can be used and a variety of techniques, most are very similar. Results from Mesotherapy can range from very good to poor, depending on the physician. Be sure the doctor you choose has received good training, has an adequate amount of experience, and is getting good results.

At the same time, success depends a great deal on the willingness of the patient. If the patient will not do what the physician advises, the patient will not see outstanding results. Compliance or noncompliance can produce dramatic differences, with a compliant patient often losing twice as much weight.

A very nice woman came into my office for her second treatment. I noticed she hadn't lost any weight or inches. I told her how unusual that was and asked if she was following a sensible diet and getting moderate exercise.

She informed me that she wasn't able to start her exercise program yet. But she excitedly reported that she was no longer eating a baked potato with her pork ribs and when she went out to eat Mexican food she no longer ate two baskets of chips with salsa. She had cut down to one!

I recalled advising her in our first meeting, as I do to all

1

of my patients, to stay away from starchy foods while taking Mesotherapy treatments. She thought *cutting back* was the same as *avoiding*. And, while I agree that cutting back is better than nothing, it's not good enough. I warned her that if she was not willing to avoid the starches, she should stop Mesotherapy. I could not, with a clear conscience, allow her to spend her money knowing that she was not going to see desirable results. Those who follow protocol will see good results, period.

Some might say that if a patient has to follow a diet, the diet is causing the loss of inches, not Mesotherapy. That is a reasonable deduction, but most of my patients who need Mesotherapy have been dieting and exercising yet still have certain fat areas they are unable to get rid of. Mesotherapy targets areas of concern, and when added to a healthy regimen, fat is reduced. But, Mesotherapy by itself is not enough; a negative calorie balance and energy exertion are required to burn fat.

A Mesotherapy injection makes fat cell walls more permeable so that fat can be released more easily, but the fat still has to be metabolized and utilized for energy. This happens when the patient exercises or her liver processes the fat and removes it from the body through normal metabolism. If neither occurs, the body will reabsorb the fat. The patient will then have the same problem she had before she started Mesotherapy.

Some people get better results from Mesotherapy treatments than others. Why? First, they do everything they can to make them work. Second, they see a physician who is familiar with both weight loss and Mesotherapy. The patient and physician can do a number of things to enhance the treatments and make them work better, which we will cover in chapters to follow. We'll start with a crash course on Mesotherapy, its full definition and history, to enhance your understanding of the process.

CHAPTER II

Definition and History of Mesotherapy

DEFINITION OF MESOTHERAPY
FOR SPOT FAT AND CELLULITE REDUCTION

Mesotherapy is a non-invasive injection therapy used to remove fat successfully exactly where you want. It is a cutting edge alternative to liposuction, plastic surgery and other invasive cosmetic procedures. This revolutionary procedure is the best treatment available for treating cellulite, and allows many women to wear shorts and swimsuits for the first time in years.

Here's what satisfied patients around the world are saying:

"I'm wearing sizes of clothes that I wore in college and I have three children now."

"My pooch is gone after 24 years."

"I have curves now that I didn't even have in college."

"I went from a size 12 to a size 8 in eight weeks."

3

HISTORY OF MESOTHERAPY

Mesotherapy, also known as Lipotherapy or nonsurgical spot fat reduction, has been touted as the latest breakthrough for body sculpting, cellulite reduction, and spot fat reduction. It is actually an aesthetic medical specialty that was developed in 1952 in Paris, France, as a treatment for pain related problems. Later it was found to be helpful for aesthetic problems such as cellulite reduction and spot fat reduction.

For years we have known that certain supplements, vitamins and/or medications taken orally can increase the body's ability to burn fat. Now, through Mesotherapy, these medications can be administered to a specific area for spot fat reduction.

Mesotherapy works by targeting receptors on the fat cell surfaces, which cause lipogenesis (fat production) and lipolysis (fat breakdown). Receptors that break down fat are known as beta receptors; receptors that create fat are alpha receptors.

Your physician will select a formula best designed to treat your condition or appearance concern. This formula is then administered through numerous microinjections into the mesoderm layer of the skin, the layer of tissue closest to the muscle, where most fat is stored. The medicine slowly diffuses into the fat cells and produces breakdown by stimulating the beta receptors and blocking absorption of the alpha receptors. The fat cell wall becomes more permeable, allowing release of the fat for use by the body.

✪ Historic overview: Basic Mesotherapy originates in the 1700s. Modern Mesotherapy takes off in 1950s. Becomes widely known and gains much respectability in 1990s.
✪ Pravaz originates injection therapy.

- ✿ 1894: Dr. Rynd uses substances at the level of the responsible nerve to treat cases of neuralgia.
- ✿ Early 1900s: Dr. Lemaire of Belgium injects procaine for neuralgia of the tri-facial nerve.
- ✿ Dr. Leriche uses intradermal injections of histamine for intercostal fractures with regression of pain.
- ✿ 1929: Dr. Sicard and Dr. Lichwitz demonstrate the role of the dermis in the treatment of visceral pain.
- ✿ 1947: Dr. Aslan introduces the use of procaine in geriatric patients.
- ✿ 1952: Dr. Pistor begins using intradermal injections of procaine on peripheral areas with positive results. Pistor publishes article titled "Brief Explanation of the Rich Properties of Procaine in Human Pathology."
- ✿ 1958: Dr. Bicheron uses injections of procaine into chronic painful spots with good results.
- ✿ Dr. Pistor and Dr. Lebel develop Lebel needle, a hollow needle 3 cm in length, very different from the 16 mm interdermic needle typical at the time.
- ✿ 1958: The name "Mesotherapy" is suggested in French medical journals. In an article published on June 4, Dr. Pistor points out the new properties of procaine and its action on tissues originating from the mesoderm being so successful, the treatment deserves the name of Mesotherapy.
- ✿ 1964: The French Society of Mesotherapy is created.
- ✿ 1976: Hospital consultations for Mesotherapy are allowed. First International Congress on Mesotherapy takes place.
- ✿ 1981: First Mesotherapy consultation for professional athletes at the Institute National de Sports de Paris is given by Dr. Jacque LeCoz.
- ✿ 1982: First university diploma in Mesotherapy is

created.

✿ June 16, 1987: French Academy of Medicine pronounces the technique of Mesotherapy an official part of traditional medicine.

✿ 1991: Dr. Pistor, now heralded as the founder of Mesotherapy, retires as head of the French Society of Mesotherapy. Dr. LeCoz assumes his position.

✿ 2003: Dr. Pistor passes away. There is much favorable publicity on CBS News and ABC News, as well as many print articles in popular women's magazines.

✿ 2004: Mesotherapy is gaining much more acceptance in the United States, with numerous national seminars.

✿ 2004: Dr. Parker speaks at the American Society of Bariatric Physicians Annual Meeting and Symposium.

CHAPTER III

What Mesotherapy Can Do for You

Mesotherapy can be used to treat almost any area of fat collection on the body, including, but not limited to, these areas or conditions:

Abdomen	Inner Thighs	Stomach Pooch
Arms	Knee Bulge	Stretch Marks
Back	Legs	Waist
Bra Bulge	Love Handles	Wrinkles
Cellulite	Saddlebags	
Double Chin	Scars	
	Skin Rejuvenation	

Probably the application of Mesotherapy that achieves the best results is spot fat reduction. It is a wonderful technique for the patient who has one or two stubborn fat areas. Although it can be used on a very overweight person, obviously a small person with limited areas of fat can lose the inches more economically than a person who has much larger areas to lose. The larger person should consider losing her extra weight before beginning Mesotherapy. Ideally, the patient will be within thirty pounds of her preferred weight before attempting Mesotherapy in conjunction with a weight loss program.

As I always tell my patients, everyone should be on a low starch and a "good fat" diet. This means avoiding the saturated and transaturated fats that are more likely to end up in arteries and intra-abdominal areas where they cause the most damage.

A second use for Mesotherapy is for cosmetic and esthetic purposes. Since Mesotherapy is an excellent technique for spot fat reduction, its cosmetic uses are almost unlimited. More and more, it is being employed for eye-pad fat.

A third application of Mesotherapy is for the face and neck areas. It is an excellent treatment for facial rejuvenation. There are a number of techniques and medications available for these treatments, which all depend on the degree of aging of the skin, the amount of wrinkles, and degree of skin laxity.

Some physicians call this a "Meso-lift," and others refer to it as "Meso-glow." Even a few doctors call it "Meso-rejuvenation." Meso-lift is not my favorite name for it because it is not a true "lift." However, it does tone up the face and gives the *appearance* of a lift in some patients. It is very good for rejuvenating the facial skin and usually gives a younger appearance. For about a week following the treatment, the patient appears to have a "youthful glow," hence the term Meso-glow, which is the name I prefer.

Mesotherapy has also been useful in treating scars. As a physician, I want to know the patient's background in relation to the treatment. The treatment of scars in people of color often makes the scarring worse instead of better. So Mesotherapy should be used cautiously on people of color and on anyone who tends to scar more severely than average.

Fifth, Mesotherapy is used for cellulite. **What is cellulite?** Cellulite is the dimpling that women around the world have grown to loathe. Cellulite occurs in the subcutaneous level of the skin. Cells are normally arranged in chambers surrounded by connective tissue much like a honeycomb. As this connective tissue contracts and hardens, it can hold the skin in place while the surrounding tissue can expand or flex with water and/or weight gain. This results in some sections of the skin being held down while others bulge: thus, dimpling.

Mesotherapy is the best treatment available for cellulite; however, in more advanced cases, it may not be enough to remove cellulite completely. Mesotherapy is most effective in the early stages; in more advanced stages of cellulite damage, Mesotherapy may not be enough. It is, nevertheless, a very helpful adjunct to other therapies. When using Mesotherapy for cellulite, it takes longer to see results as opposed to the rather quick performance seen in spot fat reduction.

Spot fat and cellulite are so common nowadays that cellulite therapy is becoming more and more sought after. I venture to say that in the future there will be very few people who haven't had a treatment at some point in their lives. Studies have reported that up to 95 percent of adult women suffer to some degree with problems of cellulite.

Reportedly, cellulite affects the self-image and self-esteem of women more than anything else. It can affect women of all ages regardless of their weight. I have seen it in women well within their target weight. Cellulite is usually found on the hips, buttocks, and thighs; however, it can appear almost anywhere. Ironically, women describe cellulite with terms of endearment such as "cottage cheese," "orange peel," and the all-time favorite, "hail damage."

Why is fat reduction so difficult for so many people, especially women? Because cells in the lower part of the body store fat more readily than the cells in the upper body, thus making weight loss in some areas almost impossible for some women. Because of this, Mesotherapy has become the preferred treatment for many women.

A sixth application of Mesotherapy is found in hair restoration. I have no personal experience in this area, and I have not heard enough positive reports from my colleagues to prompt me into trying it. I have seen cases with good results, but I don't think that the percentage of good results compares as favorably as the other areas that I have discussed. For a local area of hair loss, it can sometimes be effective, but for male pattern baldness, it takes many treatments and is not effective in most people.

Finally, Mesotherapy can be an effective treatment for pain. It can be used for sports injury therapy and athletics, rheumatology for people with arthritis, or helpful in chronic pain with any source.

In ligament repair, however, it will not cure a completely torn ligament, nor will it heal a herniated disc. Obviously, it is important to have the condition evaluated by a qualified physician to determine if you are a candidate for Mesotherapy, especially when considering it for the treatment of pain.

The advantage of Mesotherapy is that a small amount of medication can be injected into the site of the pain source and even to the area where the pain is felt. Surprisingly, that is not always the same area. For example, pain that is felt down the back of the leg actually originates from the lower back. This is usually sciatic pain, referred to as sciatica. This and similar problems can be successfully treated with Mesotherapy.

Another effective treatment for pain is **Prolotherapy** (also called sclerotherapy or ligament reconstruction). It is similar to Mesotherapy only in that it is an injection to the site of the pain. It differs greatly from Mesotherapy in its principle. Prolotherapy is useful for repairing ligaments and joints. My personal preference is to use Prolotherapy for chronic problems (problems lasting for at least six weeks) and to use Mesotherapy for acute problems (recently incurred problems) such as sports injuries.

Acute problems can also be treated with a technique called **Trigger Points.**

Additionally, **acupuncture** has been found to be effective on these acute injuries because it is used to stimulate the nerves and pathways in these areas without the use of medications.

These are the most common ways that Mesotherapy is used, and its future looks bright, with new or more refined techniques being developed continually as millions of women seek its help for spot fat reduction and cellulite.

CHAPTER IV

Chemistry Class — Mesotherapy 101

There are a number of substances that can be used in Mesotherapy, ranging from natural elements — vitamins, minerals, phospholipids, and amino acids — to a variety of drugs. Which are chosen depends on the desired results, the area to be treated, the patient's history, and physician's training. Other factors need to be taken into account also.

Many people who are doing Mesotherapy are not licensed to give medicines that are classified as drugs, so they are more likely to use homeopathic remedies. Homeopathic remedies can be very useful, but can sometimes be slower. They are usually safer than some prescribed medications.

Homeopathy was developed by a German doctor who believed that small amounts of substances could have positive effects without the danger that many drugs have. We have used this theory in our allergy practice for years by giving patients small amounts of the things they were allergic to and gradually increasing the strength. We may start with something divided 10,000 times and gradually increase the strength or dosage as the body develops immunity.

But in spot fat and cellulite reduction, patients want quick results; we don't have time for homeopathic medicine alone.

Physicians like me tend to use substances that are

natural to the body whenever possible. By "natural," I mean substances that may be found normally in the body or in the foods we eat. Some drugs may have side effects — rapid heartbeat or other unfavorable occurrences.

For spot fat reduction, one marvelous substance is **phosphatidylcholine,** which is an essential phospholipid. It occurs naturally in the body — actually makes up 50 percent or more of the cell wall. Phosphatidylcholine, a health promoting substance, usually gives the best benefits of all possible Mesotherapy ingredients. And, its safety is hard to beat; it would be exceedingly rare for someone to have an allergic reaction or toxic side effects. Only in countries outside the United States have there been reports of problems; patients were not being treated by licensed physicians or physicians were not buying phosphatidylcholine from reputable pharmacies. So please go to a properly trained physician you trust, who uses quality drugs and works in a sterile environment. A patient who employs reasonable hygiene practices should then have no reason to worry about infection.

There have been a few reported cases of arrhythmias, irregular heartbeat, most likely in persons who have been given other drugs along with phosphatidylcholine. Although the drugs are not necessary for spot fat reduction, they can in some instances speed the progress and help in cellulite reduction; thus, some doctors choose to use them.

Several university studies have proven that phosphatidylcholine does indeed work at removing fat. An obesity expert at the Baltimore VA Medical Center stated that the rate of fat breakdown increased two to three times with the use of phosphatidylcholine.

Some doctors pose the question: "What will happen to these fatty acids after they break down? Could they wind up in arteries or other tissue?" The answer is NO. Phosphatidylcholine has many health enhancing benefits other than just removing fat. Many physicians in Europe have begun to use it to treat hardening of the arteries. It is given in high doses through an IV, and it is done very safely since phosphatidylcholine is an essential phospholipid. A study reported in the journal *Atherosclerosis* showed a reduction in cholesterol, triglycerides, and LDL (bad cholesterol), and increased HDL (good cholesterol) in animals treated with essential phospholipids.

Another study showed that daily doses of essential phospholipids halted the progression of liver fibrosis. Phosphatidylcholine appears to increase the breakdown of collagen, the connective tissue protein that tends to accumulate in liver disease and promotes the scarring behind fibrosis and cirrhosis. (Remember this when we talk about treating cellulite.)

Phosphatidylcholine blocks our ability to store fat and actually increases our ability to release fat. Specifically, it is a liquid form of lecithin, naturally occurring in the body. It has been used for years to help receptor properties and accelerate lipolysis. It has this lipoytic activity by affecting the permeability of the fat cell membrane. In the United States, the injectable form of phosphatidylcholine requires a prescription.

Aminophylline is a prescription medication that is added by some physicians because it has been found to increase the lipolysis and inhibit lipogenesis. It does this by stimulating the beta receptors and inhibiting the alpha receptors.

Isoproterenol is used in localized obesity, usually below the waist. This can have cardiac effects (like stimulation) and should be used only when the patient and physician feel that it is worth the risk.

Carnitine is a natural substance that is used by the body to transport long chain fatty acids to the mitochondria of the cells where they are burned for energy. Thus, Carnitine promotes fat burning, with no side effects. Several scientific studies have shown that increased levels of Carnitine lead to increased fat burning. If you can't get fat into the mitochondria, you can't burn it off.

Carnitine is sometimes called an amino acid. This is not actually true. It is structured more like a B-vitamin. It is especially similar to choline, but Carnitine is not a true vitamin either, because the body only makes it in small amounts.

Carnitine helps to increase your metabolic rate while maintaining your muscle tissue. It is additionally useful for eliminating cravings and increasing energy.

The heart derives 70 percent of its energy from fat, and fat can't be burned without Carnitine. Carnitine is a crucial heart nutrient, and helpful in the treatment of many heart problems. It is also beneficial in lowering cholesterol and triglycerides.

Carnitine is extremely safe and highly recommended by many cardiologists, including Dr. Stephen Sinatra at the New England Heart Center, because it is known to help strengthen the heart.

Yohimbine is used by some physicians because it blocks the alpha II receptors and acts as a vasodilator, dilating blood vessels, mainly in the pelvic area; consequently it is often used in treating saddlebags. It also tends to increase sex drive.

Caffeine is a substance that is sometimes used. It acts comparably to Aminophylline as it stimulates the beta receptors.

Some physicians use **Hyaluronidase**, which acts on the connective tissue to loosen it, allowing for better diffusion of medicines. Hyaluronidase is very helpful in breaking down the fibrous bands found in cellulite.

Pentoxifylline, also known as Trentol, is commonly used for cellulite.

Mellolitis is a homeopathic preparation that acts on the microcirculation and improves lymphatic drainage — useful in cellulite problems.

Coumarin (not to be confused with Coumadin, a blood thinner) is also used by some physicians for treating cellulite.

Hyaluronic acid exists naturally in all living organisms. It is a universal component of the extra cellular space; it is a **mucopolysaccharide**. When used in Mesotherapy, it helps increase tissue hydration and cellular function. It holds more water than any other natural substance, up to 1,000 times its weight; therefore, it helps in increasing smoothness while decreasing and softening wrinkles. As a result, it is often used in the treatment of facial wrinkles.

Tretinoin stimulates the turnover of epithelial cells and repairs DNA damage — often used for facial and skin rejuvenation, stretch marks and scars.

Glycolic acid causes a local inflammation that stimulates new cell turnover and skin rejuvenation.

Many physicians will often use a multivitamin mixture along with trace minerals like zinc and selenium because they help in the rejuvenation of the skin.

Most physicians will use **lidocaine** or **procaine** as a numbing agent. This also helps to diffuse the medications they are using and spread them into the tissue better. Either will supply a vasodilating effect.

Lidocaine has replaced procaine in most treatments because there is less chance of an allergic reaction.

CHAPTER V

Frequently Asked Questions

Q: What is phosphatidylcholine?
A: Phosphatidylcholine, an essential phospholipid, is the substance most frequently mentioned in the treatment of spot fat reduction and cellulite treatment. It is the chief component in lecithin. Phosphatidylcholine has been proven to reduce cholesterol, increase metabolism, and enhance liver and other cellular functions. Lecithin has a long history of being studied extensively, over many years, and is very safe.

Q: Is phosphatidylcholine approved in all countries?
A: I cannot answer this completely. I know it is a normal substance in the body, considered a food supplement. It is present in all cells. Injections must be prescribed by a physician.

Q: How does Mesotherapy/Lipotherapy work?
A: The medication makes the fat cell membrane more permeable so that it can release the fat. After fat is released, it is utilized in the muscle for energy — burned through normal metabolism, exercise — or processed and removed from the body by the liver. The final option is for the fat to be reabsorbed by the body. This is why exercise becomes so important. Exercise will burn the fat and prohibit reabsorption. Obviously, avoiding starch and fat intake will

17

change the amount of fat available to the body and will also enhance the results.

Q: Will the solution melt other organs?
A: NO!!! This substance has been researched and used for years. There has been nothing reported (in more than fifty years of use) that would suggest this has ever happened or that there is even a remote possibility of organ damage. The basic Mesotherapy solution has been given daily in intravenous treatments with no reported organ maladies.

Q: What are the side effects?
A: When done correctly by a well-trained physician who uses sterile practices, about the only side effects are localized tenderness at the injection site, some itching, and some bruising (in those who tend to bruise easily). In the human body are many little superficial veins (and the locations of veins vary greatly from person to person), so there is a chance that the doctor may hit tiny veins and slight bruising may occur. Bruises usually disappear in a week or two. And there are substances that can be taken to minimize bruising.

An occasional lump may appear if there is bleeding under the skin. This will usually be absorbed in just a few days. Once again, it is important that the physician uses sterile techniques and the patient is careful to keep the area clean as per the doctor's instructions. I always review a list of "Do's and Don'ts" with my patients. We will discuss these later in this book.

Keep in mind that you will receive numerous tiny injections and, as a result, there will be tiny holes. You want to keep the holes free from anything that could cause an infection. Avoid hot tubs and swimming pools. They are both breeding farms for bacteria! We even prefer that you not take a sit-down bath within the first twenty-four hours after a treatment. Showers are OK, but to be safe keep all lotions, oils and soaps off the injection sites.

Q: Does it hurt?
A: You may feel *some* of the needles, but they are very small, so it is unlikely that you will feel many of them. They feel like pin pricks. We use the smallest possible needle. And we can apply a special cream ahead of time to further lessen pain. The cream partially numbs the area to be treated, taking the edge off.

Most people are just fine without the cream, though you can even take a small tube home with you if you wish. It is usually our male patients who request the cream. Men seem to be much more needle-phobic than women are.

If you decide you want to use the cream, plan to spend an extra thirty minutes in the office. This is about how long it takes the cream to take effect. Then we will proceed with your treatment.

Q: How does Mesotherapy compare to liposuction?

A: Liposuction	Mesotherapy
Quicker than Mesotherapy	Slower than liposuction
Surgical procedure	Nonsurgical procedure
Requires anesthesia	No anesthesia necessary
Takes hours to perform	Takes minutes to perform
Takes weeks to recover	No recovery time required
Can damage connective tissue	No connective tissue damage
Uneven "denting" possible	No "denting"
More likely to "dent" after weight gain	Not likely to "dent" after weight gain
Fat redeposited unevenly	Fat redeposited evenly
Can cause nerve damage	No nerve damage
Can lead to infection	No infection risk with good hygiene
Can cause death	No associated deaths reported
Cellulite waviness and skin waviness visible following	No surface irregularities or waviness visible

19

treatment	
Excessive weight loss can cause shock	Weight loss gradual and safe
Results can be unpredictable	Ninety percent success rate
Ideal for large areas of fat	Ideal for small/moderate areas of fat
Excessive swelling	Slight swelling

Liposuction has its place. It can be a very safe and effective procedure when placed in the right hands. But every surgical procedure comes with its own set of risks. It is important that you know and trust the physician, and completely understand the risks. Mesotherapy continues to gain respect and acceptability because of its success vs. risk ratio. More and more physicians are being educated and trained in Mesotherapy every year.

Mesotherapy, in general, is a much safer, more patient-friendly procedure than liposuction. Two great advantages of Mesotherapy are that it is nonsurgical, therefore not needing anesthesia, and it takes only minutes to perform. People can return to their regular daily routine immediately following a Mesotherapy treatment, where they would require up to six weeks to recover from invasive liposuction surgery. I have been told that there are as many as a hundred deaths each year as a result of liposuction, many the result of anesthesia mishaps. There have been no reported deaths with Mesotherapy.

In addition, there is a much higher chance of infection and nerve damage with liposuction. And increased chances of lumpiness or waviness in cellulite deposits. This is simply not the case with Mesotherapy. In fact, I have treated patients who had liposuction and then came to me, hoping I could smooth out the lumps liposuction created or left behind.

When a patient has liposuction, then gains weight, the fat tends to redeposit very unevenly. Ninety percent of the people who have Mesotherapy and do what they are supposed to do will get good results.

Liposuction is probably more ideal for someone who has large areas of fat to be removed. Although the safe route would be to lose the weight with diet and exercise, then remove the stubborn spot areas with Mesotherapy.

Q: How often can Mesotherapy be done?

A: Most physicians will give the treatments once a week or once every two weeks until the patient is satisfied with the results.

Q: How many treatments will it take?

A: This depends greatly on the amount of spot fat that needs to be removed, and how many areas there are. Most of our patients need five or six sessions. At the end of five sessions, the patient will then decide if they have received the desired results and are finished with treatment, or they are not quite at their goal and want to continue treatments to one or more areas, or they wish to start treatment on an area not yet treated — again employing five to six sessions.

For cellulite, most patients are going to need in the neighborhood of ten to twelve treatments.

Q: How soon will I see results?

A: For patients being treated for spot fat, *some* will see results within days; the *majority* will see a difference within two weeks. However, a *few* will take a little longer.

With cellulite, results are more gradual. Most people can tell a slight improvement by the fourth treatment. It is possible that dramatic results won't be seen until the tenth or eleventh treatment.

Q: Will the treatment cause uneven fat loss?

A: If Mesotherapy is done correctly, it should not show

uneven fat loss. I have not seen uneven loss on any of the many patients I have treated. I have had patients come to me with uneven fat loss, usually following liposuction, and we have been able to smooth it out using Mesotherapy. This normally is a concern only to patients who have experienced liposuction.

Q: Have there been any dangerous side effects reported in clinical use?

A: Dr. Patricia Rittes, who has performed tens of thousands of Mesotherapy treatments, has not come across one case with serious side effects. She reports the usual and expected side effects like bruising and itching at the site, but no unusual or risky problems.

There were some cases of severe infection and necrosis reported in Brazil from unskilled, illegal, non-clinical use, and with products that were not authorized or were expired. These incidents should not be compared to the results obtained in the sterile environment used in my office and those I would expect to find in the vast majority of offices in the United States. Again, know your physician.

CHAPTER VI

Typical Mesotherapy Sessions
in My Office

After signing in, the patient will be asked to fill out some forms. The information will give us a good idea of the patient's medical history as well as a brief family medical history. The more we know about the patient, the more precisely we can make each treatment.

We will give them some information, including media articles and other print material that will address many of the common questions about Mesotherapy. This is especially helpful to the patient who knows little or nothing about the procedure. Most of the articles we ask the patient to read are in favor of Mesotherapy; but we also provide rather rare articles that are critical. There are a very few people who can find a downside to just about anything, including Mesotherapy. Ultimately, we believe that a good patient is a well-informed patient.

Once that is accomplished, one of my nurses will take the patient to a room and talk about specific areas of concern. She will find out exactly where the patient wants the fat removed and the results expected. In order to make the patient feel completely at ease about our facility, she will explain our standards of excellence, how we do procedures in general, and the procedure being considered.

Next, the cost and payment options are discussed.

She will go over the "Do's and Don'ts" of Mesotherapy, and briefly explain the various things that can be done to ensure success. Because most women are more comfortable discussing these things with a female nurse than with a male doctor, I ask my nurses to cover this part of the consultation.

Finally, she will answer any questions up to this point.

The nurse will then bring me in and I will reinforce many of the things that my nurse just told the patient. I do this simply because a lot of information has been presented, important information, and I want to be sure everything is covered and understood. The more times someone hears something, the more likely they are to remember and understand it.

Forgive me when I, in this chapter, duplicate information found in other chapters. I want you to experience the whole process, yet some of this must be in other chapters or they would be terribly deficient.

One of the first things that I will tell a patient is that while Mesotherapy is a magnificent technique, it *is not* a miracle maker. It *is* a tool. They must have realistic expectations. We do not inject medicine into a fatty area and watch it disappear. The patient has to take an active role in making the fat go away and stay away.

I explain that when we inject an area that the patient is having trouble with, the medicine will make the fat cell walls more permeable so that the cells will release the fat more readily. Once the fat is released it will be metabolized by the liver and removed; burned up by normal metabolism, exercise, or fat-burning supplements that I offer; or reabsorbed. The key is to utilize the fat for energy.

I continue by telling them about a number of things that will make Mesotherapy work much better. One is to have a negative calorie balance, take in fewer calories than your body uses. There are those who would point out that you could lose weight anyway by doing this, and that is true, but Mesotherapy allows you to lose weight primarily from areas you target — usually the tummy, saddlebags, and thighs. Weight you haven't lost by dieting or exercise alone. Adding Mesotherapy to your diet and an exercise routine makes it much more likely that you will finally get the fat out of those stubborn areas.

Exercise has to be vigorous enough to increase your metabolism. If you do the exercise just enough to burn calories, that's good, but if you do it enough to boost your metabolism, your body will continue to burn calories for several hours after a workout, and that's great.

The next thing I will mention is that if they do everything that they should do as far as maintaining a negative calorie count, getting exercise, and taking fat-burning supplements, they will see an average of one-half inch lost per session. Those not taking all of the extra measures will notice one-fourth of an inch lost per session. If they choose to go out and eat all of the wrong things, they might even gain inches.

It is an amazing technique. Patients love it. Everyone is raving about it. But rest assured, those who are getting good results are taking responsibility for their success.

Because this is not an inexpensive procedure, it doesn't make sense to just throw your money out the window. That's exactly what you will be doing if you pay for Mesotherapy then eat and drink like you haven't a care in the world. Would you pay for a movie and then sit there with your eyes closed? No, you want to get the most for your money. Mesotherapy is the same. Watching your diet, taking the supplements, and getting some exercise is like opening your eyes at the movies!

The next thing is to decide what kind of treatment is indicated and how many treatments will be required. I will ask the patient to set a goal: an inch or two, or several inches? Most people will need five or six treatments, but that is in no way set in stone. If they are seeking cellulite reduction, they can probably double that. I always tell my patients that Mesotherapy doesn't work on everyone with cellulite. Most people are pleased with the results, though it works better on younger people and those who exercise.

Next, I cover the procedure itself. The patient will feel a little numbness and pricking sensations. They *will* feel needles, even though they are tiny. We can use numbing cream if the patient feels it is necessary. This is usually applied thirty minutes before the appointment time.

Then I tell them that they may feel tender and "prickly" for a day or two. It is not unbearable. It's just something that they are doggedly aware of.

On the first day, they will experience some itching. It is extremely important that they not scratch the area, which would increase the chances of an infection. We have never had an infected patient, but we don't want a single one. We tell them about everything that could potentially cause infection.

We go over all the above suggestions two or three times if necessary before sending the patient home. I remind them that I don't want them in a hot tub or swimming pool and to even avoid a sit-down bath. A shower is OK as long as they refrain from using soaps, lotions, and oils for twenty-four hours. I usually recommend that they take their shower or bath just before their appointment; that way they don't have to worry about it for another day. I don't want them going out in the sun or going to the tanning bed either for those first twenty-four hours.

Some people will get a little bruising, especially those people who bruise easily. A natural substance can keep bruising to a minimum. Keep in mind, bruises may be unsightly, but there is nothing harmful about them. Blood thinners like aspirin will make you more likely to bruise, so we don't recommend taking them. In fact, we don't usually treat someone taking blood thinners.

It's now time to let the patient ask any additional questions. The answers to most questions are in this book or the literature we gave at the beginning. Should they come up with unique questions, I will answer those too.

If the patient decides to do Mesotherapy, I will do a general physical, a cardiogram, and a complete blood profile. Unfortunately, if they have had these tests/exams done at another physician's office, it doesn't really help me. These tests must be performed in my office; it is of utmost importance that I make sure my patient is in good health.

There have actually been times when we discovered problems that kept us from treating a patient until they got those problems taken care of. For example, I found one woman with a goiter, which is a thyroid problem, and a couple of women with tumors in the abdomen. All three thought they were in good health. They were sent to the proper specialists. Once the problems were corrected or brought under control, we proceeded with Mesotherapy.

Once everything has been explained thoroughly and any health maladies ruled out, we can carry out the procedure as early as the next day if the lab results are back.

On treatment day, again I stress to every patient the importance of keeping the area clean, but no soaps, lotions, oils or other preparations for twenty-four hours. If they need to clean dots of blood from the site, they can use hydrogen peroxide.

I once more emphasize the importance of having a negative calorie balance. We have an outstanding weight loss program and I recommend dieting and exercise, but we don't require them.

For those who choose not to diet or don't need to lose weight, we recommend a routine of avoiding sugar, starch, alcohol, trans fats and saturated fats. I hope that after reading this book you will better understand why.

I will then remind the patient of some of the injections and natural supplements that we can offer them that support burning of fats or promote healthy liver function in general.

We also offer capsules that can help block fat and starch absorption. These last two tools are for occasional use only. They are ideal if you find yourself caught in a situation where there are no "safe" food choices. This happens at weddings, business seminars, and a variety of social parties. You are better off avoiding these situations and the foods that they invariably serve. But if you can't, these two capsules can be a lifesaver.

For example, the fat blocker can absorb the amount of fat found in one medium-sized slice of pizza. Yet if you have several slices, it won't keep you out of trouble. Common sense is still your greatest asset.

CHAPTER VII

How to Find a Mesotherapist

Nowadays, finding a Mesotherapist may be difficult. But, as time goes on, as the technique really takes off, Mesotherapists will increasingly be easier to find. The challenge then will be to find a good one who gets good results.

Word of mouth is one way to find a Mesotherapist you will be comfortable with. The more satisfied patients that he or she has, the more likely it is that word will get around. Conversely, if the practitioner has a high volume of unsatisfied patients, that news will also spread. Ideally, you will find someone you already know — a doctor or a friend who has adequate training. Most likely, you will need to put the word out to friends and co-workers. As popular as Mesotherapy is becoming, it is very likely that someone you know has had dealings with a Mesotherapist. So don't be shy about asking around.

Make sure the Mesotherapist uses good, sterile techniques. In the back of this book is a list of Mesotherapists that we have found. Most of them I know personally and can vouch for them. Some of them I don't actually know personally but have heard no negative accounts.

Right about now you may be wondering, "Can I get my personal physician to do Mesotherapy?" Absolutely, but make sure he/she gets adequate training first. I helped start the North American College of Meso-Lipotherapy so that physicians could get good training. My address and phone

29

number are listed at the back of this book under "About the Author." There are other places to be trained as well. Some are adequate — some not. Ideally, a physician would take at least one training course *and* a preceptorship. I have many physicians come to my office for a preceptorship so they can get personal attention and hands-on training.

CHAPTER VIII

Cellulite

Cellulite is possibly one of the most frightening events in the lives of many women. Probably close to 90 percent of women have cellulite to some degree. And all of them hate it.

Cellulite is a term that was coined in the early '70s to describe the dimpled appearance in the skin that many people (mostly women) have in their hips, thighs and buttocks. It is much more common in women than in men because of the differences in the way their fat layers are laid down.

For example, females have a lot more estrogen, which increases fat deposits in the thighs and lower abdominal areas especially. Females have six alpha receptors to let fat in, and only one beta receptor to let fat out. Females are also higher in alpha II in the gluteal-femoral area, while men are higher in alpha II in the abdominal area.

Cellulite is one of the biggest factors that make up a woman's self-esteem, and one of the hardest things to get rid of. Thus, billions of dollars are spent every year to eliminate cellulite. Unfortunately, much of that money is being wasted because Mesotherapy is probably the very best treatment of all.

Yet even Mesotherapy is not a cure. I stress to all of my patients that we are going to improve the appearance of cellulite in about 90 percent of patients. However, we may not get rid of it completely on but a few. If we were to grade the cellulite levels on a scale of one to ten, we can expect to improve the vast majority of patients by about 50 percent. For severe cellulite, rated ten, a patient should be happy if we could get to a five. For someone starting at five, we could expect to get her to two-and-a-half or three. So patients need to be realistic with their expectations.

It is also very important to understand that a multitude of factors are responsible for cellulite development. Therefore, the more approaches used in the treatment, the better the results. With the best approach, even the projected 50 percent can be surpassed. Though to maximize the success, a patient needs to take the extra steps along with Mesotherapy.

UNDERSTANDING CELLULITE

There have been many causes of cellulite discussed on various news programs over the years. The factors mentioned have ranged from heredity to circulation to hormone imbalance to poor diet to digestion. In this chapter I am going to cover all the factors in some detail.

If a person has a family history of cellulite, she is probably going to have it as well. However, she can stop the cellulite from getting worse or prevent its development by increasing circulation. So I believe the number one factor in preventing cellulite is increasing circulation. Conversely, decreasing circulation will accentuate it in a patient that already has cellulite.

It is important to understand how cellulite actually develops. When you have good circulation in an area of the skin — whether fat, muscles or organs — you get good oxygenation and good nutrient delivery. Everything stays healthy. Damage can result when something causes poor circulation or a buildup of toxic metabolites occurs. The factors build on each other. Toxins cause damage to the circulatory vessels. Damaged circulatory vessels can't remove toxins as usual, toxins build up, vessels are damaged even more, and the cycle continues.

This scenario applies in all aspects of circulation. Arterial circulation brings oxygen and necessary nutrients to every part of the body. Venous vessels and lymphatic vessels remove metabolites waste from all areas. When there is poor circulation and toxins build up, there is damage to the walls of the small vessels, which results in leakage into these areas. Anything that causes decreased circulation, be it in capillaries, veins or in lymphatic drainage vessels, will cause this leakage. Leakage results in highly reactive chemicals, which cause damage in the surrounding areas.

Free radicals are one of the main culprits that cause decreased circulation. Free radicals are molecules with a lone electron in the outer ring, thus very unstable, and they damage body elements they come in contact with.

When there is damage in areas predominately made up of fat cells, the result is the deposition of fibroblast cells, cells that repair tissue.

Fat cells are held together in a honeycomb-type structure, much like a beehive. Between the fat cells are little strands of fiber that give the fat cells the necessary support. Many fat cells make up your gluteal area to keep you from sitting on your tailbone.

When toxic metabolites cause leakage and inflammation, the body reacts by sending fibroblast cells that build up between the fat cells, causing thicker areas called "fibrin." These fibrin areas can distort fat cell configuration and pull down some areas of the skin. The body's lymph vessels and small capillaries are then affected, for they will be even less able to help remove pools of metabolites and the fiber buildup that causes the lumpy appearance at the surface of the skin that we call cellulite.

Without treatment, the cycle continues and it builds, eventually reaching proportions that are very noticeable "hail damage."

In order to treat and prevent cellulite we have to not only understand all the factors that contribute to poor circulation and in our treatments attack them, but also simultaneously increase the flow of blood to and from areas of concern.

What are some of the things besides *heredity* that can cause poor circulation to and from areas?

One of the main factors is a current ***medical condition***, such as obesity, diabetes and heart disease. Any person who has a tendency towards cellulite should consider being checked for these conditions and initiate preventive measures.

Yo-yo dieting is another factor that everyone should be aware of. By increasing the body weight then decreasing it quickly and repeatedly, a person causes the skin to stretch fibers in the fatty tissues, which will not always reduce back to their original size.

Obviously, a ***pregnancy*** can increase the chances of getting stretch marks resulting in skin flacidity. A woman also increases the chances of cellulite development if she gains more weight than is recommended during pregnancy or if she doesn't lose extra weight in a timely manner. The longer an area stays stretched, the less likely it will return to its original condition.

Hormones play a factor. Excess estrogen is sometimes considered a big culprit in cellulite problems. The main objective is to have a balance in the estrogen, progesterone, and other hormones in the body.

Too much ***salt*** causes the body to build up excess fluid, which can cause stretching that results in leakage into cellular tissues.

Diet is also a big factor. It is important to avoid sugar, excess trans and saturated fats, artificial sweeteners, preservatives, and food colorings. All of these can cause more free radical production in the body.

Caffeine! While it does increase metabolism in small amounts, in large amounts it increases free radical production and can cause more problems.

Smoking obviously should be avoided since cigarette smoke is one of the highest producers of free radicals, second only to radiation.

While most people don't consider *tight clothing* a health risk, it can be. Anything that restricts or interferes with the normal venous and lymphatic returns will cause more pooling in some areas. The more pooling, the higher the likelihood of fluid seeping out and causing damage.

Tight clothing can cause damage to the vessels. Lymphatic vessels and veins are not nearly as strong as arteries. Oftentimes you can actually see where tight jeans have caused pinching in certain areas. When sitting, tight jeans cause even more of a pinch in the pelvic area; a belt in the waistband will cause the jeans to tighten even more.

You may want to try this to check out my theory for yourself. Slip into a bathing suit in front of a wall mirror. Put on a tight belt. Wrap a band of cloth tightly around your abdomen and hold it or tie it there. Sit in a chair, side view in the mirror. Cross your legs. Bend forward. How do your pelvic muscles look and feel?

Although *constipation* is not generally thought of as a factor in circulation, it sometimes causes pressure in the lower pelvic area much like a fibroid tumor. Constipation may make a person more prone to poor circulation.

A *sedentary lifestyle* also causes blood to pool. The sitting position alone causes a kink in the vessels and a slowing of the blood flow.

Statistics reveal that 20 to 30 percent of the population have *food allergies or intolerances.* Most of the people are not aware of their allergies or intolerances, and fewer still know that many times these conditions will cause fluid retention and buildup resulting in irritation, increased numbers of fibroblasts, and more fibrin in areas of the body.

Alcohol is another factor that is often misunderstood. A small amount of wine, because of the high amount of antioxidants that it contains, is actually a good thing. But in larger amounts, it does more harm than good. Most other forms of alcohol are mainly harmful.

TREATMENT AND PREVENTION

Liposuction is one treatment that some people undergo for cellulite reduction, though it is not very effective. In some cases, it will temporarily make the skin appear smoother on the surface while in the long run make the condition worse. Vacuuming under the skin (an integral part of the liposuction process), actually causes irritation, damage, and additional dimpling of the skin. Scarring is also possible.

You can see that many factors are involved in treating and preventing cellulite. Let's talk a little bit about some of the things that you can do along with the Mesotherapy to help make it work better.

Anything that increases the circulation will help. In general, the more exercise you do, the better. Extreme exercising can sometimes aggravate a condition, but few people have that problem.

The best exercises move the leg muscles to increase circulatory flow. Swimming is a very valuable exercise for this purpose. Walking and jogging are both good, as well.

I highly recommend some specific exercises because I have found them to be greatly effective in increasing the venous and lymphatic return flow. One of these is deep breathing. Try this: Take a deep breath and feel your diaphragm push down into your belly. You will see your belly bulge out. Practice it this way at first. This helps to determine if you are getting a good, deep breath. Once you are comfortable with this, then it will be helpful to occasionally take a deep breath and push the belly down while holding the belly in. This causes even more pressure that is negative and helps with the return flow.

A second exercise you can try is leg raises — also called calf-raises. One of my favorites is a technique that ballet dancers use. Walk around on your tiptoes. You will feel this in your calf muscles. While it sounds simple enough, you will find that it is difficult to do for very long periods. Eventually you will be able to increase the amount of time you can spend on your toes. Women should do this exercise frequently. You might have noticed that ballet dancers have far fewer problems with cellulite than the general public.

Sit-ups are very good because they help to tone up the abdominal muscles and aid the movement of fluid from the pelvic area.

A fourth exercise worth mentioning is one that I call "The Belly Button Exercise." For this one, you concentrate on your belly button, trying to suck it into your spine, hold it for a second or two, relax, and repeat. This is an excellent exercise to help the return flow of the circulatory system.

You need to work continuously to halt the cycle of cellulite buildup by getting good circulation regularly. And you have to have a good, nutritious diet. Like a good diet, cellulite exercises are not something you can do one week, skip the next week, have another good week, then take another week off.

As with anything in life, your sins will add up, whether severe cellulite was caused at one time in your life or slowly over a lifetime. The sad fact is that some of the problem areas will become permanent and irreversible. But, on a happy note, if we get at it early we can help improve it a lot. Even then, the patient has to work continuously to keep it from building up again. Just keep reminding yourself of the things you need to do to prevent further development of cellulite and stay positive.

A number of supplements are helpful in the mobilization and removal of fat. Numerous supplements help with circulation. Several stimulate burning of fat by affecting the beta cells that help cause lipolysis of fat. If you are interested in knowing more about these, contact my office listed in the "About the Author" page at the back of this book.

Some authorities have proposed a number of new massage-type treatments, and they can be helpful to a degree. Massage itself is helpful in increasing circulation to and from key areas as long at it is not too vigorous. Keep in mind that aggressive massaging can damage small venous and lymphatic vessels. Machines at the forefront of this technology — Endermologie, rolling cylinders, and sucking machines — may to a degree help in some cases as long as there is no damage to the vessels.

With my patients, we use Mesotherapy ingredients that do a multitude of things, like increase circulation, improve venous and lymphatic drainage, help dissolve fat, and increase the thermogenesis, or burning, of fat.

We also use lipotropic injection and AMP injections that we will discuss later. Just remember that the lipotropic injection helps the liver process and remove fat, and the AMP injection helps in the burning of fat. The idea is to cooperate with and encourage the "good fats," the essential fatty acids that help with mobilization and proper metabolism of fats.

We ask our patients to follow a good diet, do the suggested exercises, and drink lots of healthy liquids. We have found that it is very useful to have a water intake of at least sixty-four ounces per day. I recommend this helpful formula (as part of your sixty-four ounces per day) so patients can better avoid sodas: four ounces of cranberry or grape juice mixed with about twenty-eight ounces of water.

One other supplement that we use is proteolytic enzyme, under the brand name Prevenzyme. It contains a concentration of enzymes that help with the breakdown and removal of toxins and waste products in the body.

For people who have a tendency toward fluid retention we recommend a supplement called Rodex Forte. We use it because it contains a special form of B-6 that acts as a natural diuretic. We do not want to use any kind of regular water pill that could cause an electrolyte imbalance, thus doing more harm than good.

By using these techniques along with Mesotherapy, there is hope that cellulite can be controlled. As with spot fat reduction, there is no miracle cure, but there is an answer.

I do want to add that it is important that you do these things to prevent more buildup of cellulite. I have had patients who have done all of these things without Mesotherapy and they did not get good results. With Mesotherapy, they found improvement. Some of them questioned the "extra" things because they didn't seem to help before. My explanation was always that Mesotherapy makes all of these things more likely to work. Without them, not only will the Mesotherapy work less effectively, but also the cellulite will return or build up in the future.

CHAPTER IX

Injections and Supplements
Used to Enhance Mesotherapy

INJECTIONS

Adenosine monophosphate (AMP) causes fat cells to release their stored fat so it can be burned as energy. This process happens in the Krebs Cycle (energy cycle) in the body. Studies show that in most obese people, there is not enough AMP in the cycle to initiate fat burning. Increasing the amount of AMP in the body increases the fat burning.

Mitochondria are small "furnaces" present in every cell in your body. Studies suggest that mitochondria function inefficiently in most people, especially in obese people and those who suffer from chronic fatigue. Almost 90 percent of the energy that you need for metabolism, development, and life itself is produced in mitochondria. If functioning improperly, they are not burning fat sufficiently and not producing energy efficiently.

Certain things are essential for the body's energy transport system to do its job of harvesting more than 75 percent of the ATP energy from food. Some necessary substances are ATP, Coenzyme Q10 (CoQ10), acetyl-L-carnitine, B complex, and adenosine — the main useable form of ATP.

AMP has an effect on the cellular level. It has been hypothesized that giving AMP, which converts to ATP in the body, increases the calories burned by pumping sodium and potassium across cell membranes. Study data shows that within an hour of injecting 25 mg of AMP into a patient, 90 percent of it had been converted to ATP.

People receiving AMP should notice a subtle increase in energy. It is not felt as a "nervous energy" like one would expect if they were to take a stimulant. Instead, it tends to increase endurance. Patients notice that before they started taking AMP injections they would "run out of gas" at the end of the day. After taking AMP they found themselves continuing activities much longer than they were able to before.

We have been using this product for about twenty years, and although we haven't found it to be a miracle, it has been extremely effective in boosting metabolism, energy and overall weight loss. Because energy levels improve as the metabolism is boosted, we encourage chronic fatigue sufferers to utilize the AMP injection as well.

Lipotropic nutrients are compounds that promote the flow of fat and bile from the liver. In essence, they produce a "decongesting" effect on the liver and promote improved liver function and fat metabolism.

Methionine is one of the sulfur-containing amino acids (cysteine and cysine are others) and is important for many bodily functions. It acts as a lipotropic agent (like inositol and choline) to prevent excess fat buildup in the liver and other body parts. Methionine is helpful in relieving or preventing fatigue, and may be useful in some allergy cases because it reduces histamine release. Methionine works as an antioxidant (free radical deactivator) through conversion to L-cysteine in order to neutralize toxins.

Inositol, a nutrient belonging to the B vitamin complex, is closely associated with choline. It aids in metabolism of fats and helps reduce blood cholesterol. Inositol participates in the action of serotonin, a neurotransmitter known to control mood and appetite.

41

Choline is considered one of the B-complex vitamins as well as a lipotropic nutrient. It is present in the body of all living cells and functions with inositol as a basic constituent of lecithin. Choline appears to be associated with the utilization of fats and cholesterol in the body. It prevents fats from accumulating in the liver and facilitates metabolism and removal. It is essential for the health of the liver and kidneys.

The biggest problem with losing weight is getting fat out of the cell and into the liver where it can be converted into energy. That is the purpose of the lipotropic injection.

Nutrition-oriented physicians use lipotropic formulas to treat a wide variety of conditions, including liver disorders, hepatitis, cirrhosis, chemical induced liver disease, and weight management.

SUPPLEMENTS

Sources for all of the following supplements can be found at the end of this book in Appendix 2.

AMP and Lipotropic are available in a pill form. While they are not quite as effective as the injections, they are still very helpful.

Calcium/magnesium (with natural vitamin D). Studies have shown that when the diet is high (1,000 mg or higher) in calcium, more body fat is lost. Dieting can deplete the body of calcium, which can lead to osteoporosis and osteoarthritis. It can also pull the color and strength from your teeth. Whole milk is high in fat, and you do not want to add the 200-300 calories that four or five glasses of milk would add to your daily caloric intake; therefore, a calcium supplement or skim milk is preferable.

It is important that you take calcium with magnesium and with natural vitamin D to help distribute the calcium properly. It is important to get the calcium into the bones and teeth rather than the joints and arteries, which is a possibility if you are in the majority of people who do not properly metabolize calcium on your own.

Studies have shown another form, calcium pyruvate, is also very effective, increasing fat loss up to 48 percent. These studies, done at the University of Pittsburgh School of Medicine, have prompted me to start using this form of calcium on many of my patients.

Carbohydrate blocker. The American diet is mainly made up of potatoes, rice, pasta, and breads (complex carbohydrates). In fact, an average American gets one-half of their total calories from these complex carbohydrates.

During the digestive process, the body converts complex carbohydrates into sugar. If these sugar molecules aren't burned off through exercise, they can lead directly to an increase in fat mass. The body is storing these fat molecules for future use. Over time, an inactive lifestyle can cause the stored fat to accumulate and a substantial weight gain is the result.

The carbohydrate blocker is a safe and effective way to reduce the conversion of starch to sugar and then into fat. It actually neutralizes the digestive enzyme, alpha amylase, produced in the pancreas, before starch can be converted into sugar. Carbohydrates simply pass through the digestive tract, reducing the amount of calories absorbed.

This supplement is not for everyday use — occasional use is best. If a patient needs the supplement daily, this means she is eating foods that are a detriment to her weight loss regimen. While this product can *help* to make up for some of the evils of eating carbohydrates occasionally, it cannot possibly make up for frequent consumption.

The active ingredient is a concentrated extract of the white kidney bean. This is a natural, non-stimulant, dietary supplement, but do not take this supplement if you are allergic to kidney beans.

L-Carnitine can help you lose weight, increase energy, and support heart health. L-Carnitine is a water-soluble nutrient found in all living tissue; its chief role is to create energy. Since energy is produced in mitochondria, no matter how much you diet or exercise, if fat isn't getting into mitochondria it is not being burned off. L-Carnitine does just that! It transports fat into mitochondria so the fat can be burned off and become energy your body needs to generate, defend, and restore cell membranes, enabling them to better fight viruses and bacteria.

L-Carnitine also helps increase the metabolic rate while maintaining muscle tissue. This is very important because most of the fat burning takes place in the muscles. L-Carnitine promotes liver health, and because the liver is the detoxifier for the body, it is crucial that the liver functions optimally. Additionally, studies have shown that L-Carnitine is an important nutrient for keeping blood sugar constant; therefore, it improves insulin sensitivity.

Researchers believe more and more that the aging process begins in the mitochondrion. As we age, energy production is less efficient due to impaired or damaged mitochondria. Unrestrained free radicals break down cell membranes, causing cell functions to be interrupted. If your mitochondria are healthy, so are you.

If you want your garden to grow and thrive, you have to give it proper nutrients and make sure it is tended properly for a fine crop of fruits and vegetables. Mitochondria are much the same. If you want them to continue to burn fat for you and give you the energy you need, you must give them proper nutrients. CoQ10 and L-Carnitine are two of the best nutrients that you can provide to the mitochondria. L-Carnitine is found in red meat, but you would have to eat pounds of red meat daily to get enough. The best way to receive optimal benefits of L-Carnitine is to take a high

44

quality L-Carnitine supplement. The average recommended dose of L-Carnitine when combined with a sensible diet and moderate exercise is up to 2,000 mg per day. The average adult gets about 50-100 mg per day through food intake, and only about 65 to 75 percent of that is actually absorbed.

L-Carnitine comes in many forms. Some forms have better bioavailability (the amount of a nutrient that actually is delivered to your tissues) than others.

Once again, just a few of the many reasons to take L-Carnitine: increase fat burning, increase energy, lower cholesterol, lower triglycerides, promote heart health, reduce food cravings, promote good circulation, promote liver health, increase sports endurance, and help chronic fatigue symptoms.

Fat blocker: Chitosan, Rhosiola Rosea and vitamin C. Combined in proper proportions, the fat blocker can help minimize the damage done when eating high-fat foods. This natural supplement is similar to the once popular drug Xenical. It has the ability to absorb fourteen times its weight in dietary fat, keeping it from entering the bloodstream by soaking it up and passing it out of the body before it has the chance to be converted into body or arterial fat. It also facilitates the release of excess fat from the adipose tissue and allows stored fatty acids to be available for immediate energy use. This natural fat absorber does not have to warn its consumers of possible undesirable, uncontrollable "events" like its expensive prescription counterpart does. The natural form is usually only a problem in people allergic to shellfish and/or iodine.

Like the carbohydrate blocker, we do not recommend this product for everyday use, but it is a wonderful tool for that occasional circumstance when good food choices are just not possible. It seems that every season comes with its own set of unavoidable situations. Summer brings weddings, vacations, and baseball games. Autumn, of course, brings Thanksgiving. Winter wiles you with Christmas gatherings and New Year's parties. Spring lures you with Valentine's Day candies, Spring Break activities, graduation celebrations, and that long-awaited outdoor barbecue. As you see, there will always be something trying to trip you up. The best line of defense is to avoid as many tricky situations as possible. The next best thing is to make good choices when they are offered. The final option is to take all the precautions that you can: a safe fat absorber, along with a good carb-blocker. People who are allergic to shellfish or iodine should not take chitosan.

Chromium plays a crucial role in weight control. It is required for normal protein, fat, and carbohydrate metabolism. It is important for energy production — can even help regulate appetite. It reduces sugar cravings by helping insulin to control blood sugar, thus reducing the highs and lows of sugar levels and cravings. Chromium increases lean body mass while decreasing fat mass. Chromium is a natural and necessary cofactor of insulin, which cannot perform its vital functions without chromium.

Why do I keep stressing insulin and nutrients that affect insulin? Insulin has an undeniably important role in the human physiology. Insulin promotes the uptake of glucose in cells. It is necessary to the metabolism of fat and protein; it enhances the brain uptake of tryptophan for appetite control. Insulin reduces the output of free fatty acids from adipose tissue and increases the metabolic rate. This is a big role for one hormone to play, but given the right nutrients, insulin will continue to do its job well. Without proper care, insulin can become very hard to manage. And how we treat our body now dictates how it will treat us later in life.

Studies reveal that 96 percent of the people tested were deficient. And 90 percent of those eating an average American diet received less chromium chromate than the government's recommended daily allowance (RDA). Not one person in the study met the minimum RDA of chromate. Why are Americans deficient in chromium? Plant foods are a poor source of chromium. This is because there is not enough of it in the agricultural soil. Chromium is not essential to plant life; it is essential only to human life.

We are deficient also because of food processing, canning, freezing, blanching, and the adding of preservatives. Commercial food treatments all cause food to have even smaller amounts of chromium than they already have.

Baked products have no chromium; these include crackers, bread, pastries and pasta made with white flour. Eating chocolate, ketchup, sweets, desserts, sodas and other foods high in simple sugars can cause chromium losses of up to 300 percent. The American diet is a dangerous diet.

Chromium comes in two major forms. Picolinate is the most commonly used form; chromate is the most effective form. Because it is more efficient at helping insulin, we recommend chromium chromate to our patients.

Special blends of fiber and herbs. At my office we offer a unique blend of fiber and herbs designed to provide bulk in the diet and cleanse the lower intestine and colon. The product contains Black Walnut, Burdock Root, Echinacea, Fennel Seed, Guar Gum, Licorice Root, Oat Bran Fiber, Papaya Parsley, Psyllium Seed Hulls, and Rhubarb Root. In addition, the herbs absorb toxins in the digestive tract. The ingredients work together to kill and expel parasites, promote weight loss, purify the blood, help digestion, fight infection, and normalize appetite. Royal Nutrition makes this particular blend.

The liver is the main organ for fat metabolism and detoxification in your body. If the liver is busy with detoxification, it is less able to work as well at fat metabolism, so anything that helps detoxify the body will automatically help fat metabolism.

Green Tea. Also known as camellia sinensis, green tea has been used for stomach disorders, vomiting, diarrhea, excessive cholesterol levels, cancer reduction, and as an antioxidant. But the main reason we use it with Mesotherapy is because it increases metabolism and fat burning.

Omega-3 fatty acids are the most important essential nutrient that is almost entirely missing from our diets today. There is now overwhelming evidence from thousands of clinical studies that show Omega-3 fatty acids can improve health and help prevent disease — including lowering triglycerides, promoting general heart benefits, and improving brain function. Eating fish such as salmon, cod, and mackerel, as well as taking fish oil supplements, can be an effective therapy.

One study even showed that a daily fish oil supplement may help heart attack survivors reduce their risk of sudden death by as much as 42 percent.

Because our bodies cannot produce or manufacture their own essential fatty acids, they must be obtained from specific foods or supplements. The first two acids in a typical Omega-3 pill are **EPA** (eicosapentaenoic acid) and **DHA** (docosahexaenoic acid). Both are found in cold-water fish. Fresh seaweed is the only known plant food that contains much EPA or DHA. The third type of Omega-3 fatty acid is called **ALA** (alpha-linolenic acid), found in flaxseeds, dark-green leafy vegetables, and some vegetable oils. Although it is possible to get EPA and DHA from plant seed oils, such as flaxseed, chances are that you are not getting enough of these valuable substances even if you take flaxseed oil daily! Why? Because the Omega-3s in flaxseed oil and other plant oils do not contain DHA and EPA, although they do contain the precursor to DHA and EPA in the form of ALA.

In order for your brain and heart to get the benefit of EPA and DHA, your body must be capable of converting the ALA to DHA and EPA. Unfortunately, unless all your organs are functioning smoothly, this conversion more than likely will not happen. Even if your body is in peak condition, you will convert less than 20 percent of the ALA to DHA and EPA. Therefore, the only way to ensure that you get enough of these essential nutrients is by taking fish oil supplements.

As far as weight loss is concerned, people taking fish oil while following a supervised diet tend to lose weight more efficiently. Fish oil also lessens side effects of weight loss such as hair loss and dry skin. Fish oil has the ability to affect a group of hormones called cytokines. In particular, a cytokine known as the tissue necrosis factor (TNF) is considered one of the molecular causes of insulin resistance and the corresponding increase in insulin levels. Basically, people with insulin resistance tend to eat too much; their insulin levels stay elevated in the bloodstream, which drives down blood sugars, making them hungrier.

Hydroxycitric acid or "Bio-Citrin" is for people who need help with appetite control. Garcinia cambogia, an herbal extract, is one of the safest appetite suppressants that you can obtain without a prescription.

Research suggests that it not only suppresses appetite, but reduces the conversion of carbohydrates into stored fat. A study published in the *International Journal of Obesity* in 1996 reported that patients on a 1,200-calorie diet with 1.3g of hydroxycitric acid per day lost an average of fourteen pounds in a two-month period. People on the same diet taking a placebo lost only an average of eight pounds.

Prevenzyme is a proteolytic enzyme that can naturally reduce inflammation, which retards the healing process and makes it more likely for fibroblasts to build up, causing cellulite. Proteolytic enzymes can be helpful in preventing cellulite formation and hopefully break down the fiber bands found in cellulite. Proteolytic enzymes will neutralize braykinins and proinflammatory icosinoids to levels where synthesis, repair and regeneration occur naturally. Proteolytic enzymes can be taken on an empty stomach so they will not be used up in digestion. When taken with food, they will work mainly on digesting the food.

Pituitary. We use a sublingual tablet of a homeopathic preparation made from the pituitary gland that is excellent at helping to make fat more likely to come off hip and thigh areas. Several years ago at a weight loss seminar, a gray-haired physician told me that if I started offering these little tablets to my female patients I would have them as patients for life. And he was pretty close on that one. Women love having slim hips and thighs.

Carniforskolin contains two products that enhance lean body mass, decrease fat, and increase energy. Forskolin is an adenylate cyclase activator (the enzyme involved in the production of cyclic AMP). Pharmacologic studies indicate that forskolin shifts the proportion between lean body mass and fatty tissue in favor of lean body mass. The effect can be measured by decreases in the waist-hip ratio and the body mass index. It is believed to increase thyroid function, regulate insulin secretion, and aid in metabolism of carbohydrates, fats, and proteins.

Acetyl-L-carnitine assists in the transport of fat through cell membranes and into mitochondria, where fats are metabolized to produce cellular energy — ATP. Since acetyl-L-carnitine is also an excellent heart and brain nutrient (increasing short- and long-term memory), I have all of my heart patients taking it.

Healthy Aging Formula is a product that I think everyone over the age of 30 should be taking. Since research has suggested that levels of DHEA and 3-Beta (3B-acetoxyandrost-5-ene-7,17-dione), a natural metabolite of DHEA, decline as we age, and DHEA converts to sex hormones (testosterone and estrogen), there are safety concerns that 3-Beta relieves, without the worry of getting sex hormones that are not needed. Because 3-Beta does not convert into sex hormones, it allows people to safely recapture the enjoyment and quality of life they had when they were young.

Another benefit of this formula is weight loss. In a random study reported in *Current Therapeutic Research*, patients taking 3-Beta lost three times more weight and body fat over an eight-week study.

And the formula contains a bioactive, hyperimmune, milk protein concentrate that lowers inflammation — very effective in people with arthritis and fibromyalgia. Remember the inflammation and laying down of fibroblasts in cellulite that we talked about?

Hoodia gordonii may be one of the most powerful appetite suppressants available. African bushmen used this substance to give themselves energy during long hunting trips. Hoodia curbs the appetite while providing energy and alertness without the nervous jitters that most diet drugs cause.

A fifteen-day study conducted in Leicester, England, divided morbidly obese patients into two groups. One group was given Hoodia gordonii. The other, a placebo. Both groups were kept in closed quarters, only able to read and watch television. By the end of the study, the Hoodia gordonii group had reduced their caloric intake by one thousand calories per day.

You may begin to see more advertisements for Hoodia gordonii in the near future, but be sure you buy it from a reputable source. Many sources do not provide a good quality product or provide only a fraction of the strength needed. In the back of this book you will find the address of a supplier that will provide a quality product at a fair price. Of course, it is not the only good company out there.

MESOTHERAPY STUDIES

A major study on Mesotherapy for fat reduction for cosmetic purposes was reported in 1998 at the 5th International Meeting of Mesotherapy in Paris, France.

Italian physician Sergio Meggiori presented his work with phosphatidylcholine in the treatment of xanthelasmas, though his research at that time was in the use of phosphatidylcholine for other health problems as well as spot fat reduction.

In 1989, Bobkova published a study in *Kardiologiia* on the metabolic effect of Lipostable Forte, a brand name of phosphatidylcholine. The summary stated that phosphatidylcholine improved the cell membrane receptor properties and increased sensitivity to insulin and accelerated lipolysis.

A VA study in the United States showed the most common cocktail with phosphatidylcholine actually increased the rate of fat burning by two to three times.

There was an interesting study by Glynis Ablon, M.D., and Adam Rotunda, M.D., of UCLA reported in 2004 in the *American Society for Dermatoligic Surgery* on the use of phosphatidylcholine for treatment of the lower eyelid fat pads. Adam Rotunda, whom I have visited with at various meetings, reported that 80 percent of the patients got good results with these treatments.

Dr. Patricia Rittes of Brazil has reported on a study that consisted of four of these treatments per patient. The result was a clear improvement in all patients. She also reported that there was no return of the local fat as long as there was weight gain of no more than four kilograms. This was reported in both *The Plastic Surgery Magazine* and *American Society for Dermatologic Surgery.*

My study for the North American College of Mesotherapy followed fifty patients receiving spot fat reduction in the abdominal area. They were followed for six weeks and received one treatment each week for the first four weeks.

The patients were measured before the first treatment at the naval, two inches above the naval, and two inches below the naval. They were measured again two weeks after their last treatment.

The same medicine was used in all fifty patients. The patients were encouraged to avoid sugar and starchy foods, as well as trans and saturated fats — although avoidance was not required. All patients were encouraged to exercise regularly — once again, not required.

The average change was 3.34 inches, with a low of 1 inch to a high of 8 inches. This range can be explained because a strict diet and exercise were not mandatory. The patients who followed a smart diet and exercised obviously got better results.

Another item worth noting is a patient who was featured on the local evening news in my hometown. The NBC affiliate has a feature they call *Does It Work?* In each segment they choose a product or service and take it to various members of the community to find out if it does what it says it will do. The producers asked me to consider letting them come in and take photos of a patient before, during, and after treatment. I was hesitant because some programs have a tendency to make things like Mesotherapy look bad. But after meeting with the reporter and the producer, I decided I was secure enough about their integrity, that they truly wanted to know if it works and was it a newsworthy subject. I felt so strongly about the positive results of Mesotherapy that I thought it was worth my time.

My next concern was, "Who will the patient be?" I was worried that if the patient chose to not follow all of the recommendations for enhancing Mesotherapy that the results would not be terrific. If results were just so-so, it would be a black mark on my reputation and the field of Mesotherapy. After talking with the patient they chose, I decided that she would probably do what I was going to request of her and would be a good patient. So I agreed to the challenge.

She was 33, had lost most of her excess weight after multiple pregnancies, but still had that "baby pooch" in her stomach. We were happy to treat her. All we asked was that she watch her starches and fats, and get regular exercise.

She received six treatments over a course of eight weeks. Her waist at the beginning was 35½ inches. At the end it was 29¾. She was delighted and we were relieved.

When the reporter and producer returned to record the results, they were amazed. They rate results from zero to four stars. Zero going to a product that just didn't deliver, and a four going to a product that did what it said it would do and more. We were thrilled to be among the very few recipients of four stars.

CHAPTER X

Understanding Sugar and Starches

Whenever your blood sugar level drops, you crave food — especially starches and sweets. When you give in to these cravings and eat them, your blood sugar rises. Your pancreas releases insulin to lower your sugar. Then the cycle starts all over again.

The pancreas breaks the starches and sweets down to glucose, which is converted to triglycerides and stored in fat tissue if it is not used for energy. Therefore, it is extremely important that you keep your blood sugar at a steady, normal level. The best way is to not go long periods without eating, and eat more protein, complex carbohydrates, and fiber.

University of Illinois researchers found that increasing protein in the diet stabilizes blood sugar through the action of the amino acid leucine. Leucine exerts a short-term inhibition of new sugar production by the liver.

Foods that have complex carbohydrates such as beans, fruits and vegetables break down slowly in your body, thus avoiding the sugar spikes and fat deposits that follow. They also prevent the cycle:

low sugar => cravings => high sugar =>
fat deposits => low sugar => cravings =>
etc.

Sodas, juices, sweets, cakes, cookies, and chips are absorbed so rapidly that insulin turns on the fat production and turns off the fat burning. You may get a brief surge in energy, but when this sugar rush is over, you're more tired, depressed and irritable.

Don't rely on the net carb numbers; they can give you a false sense of security. A light beer (3 net carbs) or a bag of low-carb chips (4 net carbs) will cause many more problems than an apple, at about 17 net carbs.

Eating three smaller meals and two to three healthy snacks each day, with a small amount of protein or complex carbohydrates, will keep your sugar levels more stable and help prevent cravings. This is easy to do for most people — just have a few nuts or a few wedges of an apple, orange, pear, peach or nectarine between meals.

Spreading the food out also keeps your metabolism up so you will continue to burn fat. Going long periods without eating actually causes your metabolism to slow down, which is how a bear survives long periods of hibernation.

And remember, eat protein. It builds muscle and your body puts out more energy (burns more calories) to maintain muscle than it does to maintain fat. The higher the percentage of muscle mass in your body, the higher your metabolic rate or metabolism. If you have excess body fat, increasing muscle mass by exercising and following a high protein diet will increase your metabolism and help to burn your body's fat calories.

WHAT ABOUT LIQUOR, WINE AND BEER?

Studies have shown that drinking small amounts in moderation is not nearly as much a problem as is drinking large amounts on weekend outings. Many people, especially young people, tend to stay away from alcohol during the week and then overindulge on weekends.

A University of Buffalo study confirmed that drinking a small amount consistently, like a glass of wine or one beer each day, causes a much lower fat gain than binge drinking, even if the amount of total alcohol consumed is the same. The study further revealed that liquor is the most damaging, wine is next, and beer the least harmful.

Below is a list of popular libations and their carbohydrate counts. You will notice a dramatic difference between products.

Popular Brews and Their Carb Counts

Beer	Carbs per bottle
Rock Green Light Low Carb	2.4g
Michelob Ultra Low Carb	2.6g
Aspen Edge Low Carb	2.6g
Miller Lite	3.2g
Amstel Light	5.0g
Coors Light	5.0g
Bud Light	6.6g
Heineken	9.8g
Budweiser	10.6g
Coors	11.3g
Michelob Light	11.7g
Rolling Rock	13.0g
Miller Genuine Draft	13.1g
Guinness	17.6g
Zima	30g

Wine

Most wine coolers and hard ciders will be 26 grams and higher.

CHAPTER XI

Understanding Fat Metabolism

Many people have the false perception that all fats are bad. Actually, a certain amount of fat in the diet is necessary for you to absorb fat solulable vitamins, and fats supply the essential fatty acids that are so necessary to the body. They are also necessary for producing hormones, cushioning vital organs, forming the myelin sheaths around neurons, and producing energy.

Since the liver handles most of the fat metabolism, it is important to keep it healthy. And since the liver is the main organ for detoxification, don't overload your body with toxic poisons that can overwork or damage it. Poisons range from air pollutants (auto exhaust and cigarette smoke), poisons on or in our food (pesticides and synthetic hormones), and things you drink (alcohol, for instance).

Treat your liver right and it will do a much better job of removing fat for you. We often see people with high liver enzymes (indicating liver damage) that come back to health after establishing a healthy diet.

The most plentiful fats in your body are triglycerides. There are natural substances that help your body metabolize triglycerides better, such as the Omega-3 fatty acids.

Two things to remember: When you eat protein and carbohydrates, your metabolism tends to burn up fat first, whereas the rest of your body tends to think fat is to be stored until needed. In addition, an excess of anything —

carbohydrates, fat, or protein — will eventually be converted to triglycerides and stored as fat.

CHAPTER XII

Fast Foods

Fast foods typically contain high amounts of trans fats, saturated fats, starches and sugars — in increasingly larger portions. Studies have shown that adolescent girls who ate fast foods four or more times a week consumed about 185 to 260 calories per day more than those who did not. Eating dinner with one's family seems to improve diet quality with fewer saturated and trans fats, fewer sugars (especially from soft drinks), but more fresh fruits and vegetables.

The Centers for Disease Control (CDC) estimates that 64 percent of Americans are overweight; this is the highest amount ever. In addition, obesity has now overtaken smoking as the leading preventable cause of death. If you won't do it for yourself, do it for your children. The rate of obesity in children has doubled, and one out of three children will now probably develop diabetes in their lifetime since children tend to adopt their parents' bad habits.

CHAPTER XIII

Sensible Diet for Mesotherapy

If you have a favorite diet of your own, just follow it. But be sure to avoid sugar, starches, trans fats and saturated fats. Avoid salt and sodas as well.

If you would like to follow my preferred diet, use the following menu as a guide. Remember that you should never begin a weight loss or workout program without first consulting your physician.

BREAKFAST
1. 8 oz. skim milk OR 1 cup of low-fat yogurt
2. Choose ONE of the following:

1 apple	1 medium size wedge of watermelon
1 poached egg	1 medium size wedge of cantaloupe
1 peach	1 pear
1 nectarine	1 unripe banana (limit 2 per week)
½ grapefruit	1 orange
1 cup of melon cubes	
2 medium size wedges of honeydew	

MID-MORNING SNACK
½ piece of fruit from list above
3-4 nuts: Brazil nuts, peanuts, walnuts or almonds

LUNCH
4 oz. meat <u>AND</u> 2 cups of
cooked vegetables (see list on page 63)
An unlimited amount of uncooked vegetables from
vegetable list can be eaten.

MID-AFTERNOON SNACK
½ piece of fruit from list on previous page
3-4 nuts: Brazil nuts, peanuts, walnuts or almonds

SUPPER
6 oz. meat (see list below) <u>AND</u>
2 cups of cooked vegetables (see list on page 63)
An unlimited amount of uncooked vegetables from
vegetable list can be eaten.

MID-EVENING SNACK
½ piece of fruit from list on page 61
3-4 nuts: Brazil nuts, peanuts, walnuts or almonds

<u>MEATS</u>

The following meats may be eaten in these proportions:
4 oz. at lunch   ***   6 oz. at supper

extra lean	turkey	sirloin steak
ground beef	salmon	T-bone steak
pot roast	tuna	round steak
beef hearts,	cod	filet mignon
liver or kidney	bass	2 eggs
lamb kidney	flounder	
chicken	haddock	

VEGETABLES

When uncooked, the following vegetables
may be eaten in unlimited amounts.
When cooked, 2 cups at lunch and
2 cups at supper.

green beans	green bell peppers	garlic
broccoli	lettuce	spinach
cabbage	asparagus	tomatoes
celery	Brussels sprouts	radish
cucumbers	okra	

OTHER REALLY IMPORTANT INFORMATION

Unlimited amounts of water and tea are allowed. Diet sodas and other sugar-free drinks are allowed only occasionally. Alcohol and regular sodas should be absolutely avoided.

Do not overuse salt. One-fourth teaspoon of extra salt can cause one-half a pound of water retention. If water retention becomes an issue for you, it is of utmost importance that you use water pills or diuretics *only* under the careful supervision of a physician. We offer a safe, natural supplement for water retention called Rodex Forte.

In this book I will say this a number of times, but it cannot be stressed enough: Never start this or any other diet or a new or enhanced exercise program without the continued supervision of a physician.

CHAPTER XIV

Exercise for Fat Loss

Following a sensible diet and exercising can double the results you see with Mesotherapy. The best exercise to increase your metabolism is either weight lifting or aerobic exercise.

You don't have to lift very heavy weights. But because muscle takes more calories to maintain, the more muscle you have, the more calories your body burns when at rest.

When I recommend aerobic exercise, I'm not saying that you have to do a Jane Fonda program or "Sweatin' to the Oldies" — although you can if you want. What I am recommending is that you do some activity that is vigorous enough to get your heart rate up and keep it up for at least thirty minutes. Now, if you haven't been exercising regularly, don't start your exercise regimen on the first day with the thirty minutes I just suggested. Instead, work your way to thirty minutes gradually. To get even better results, exercise twice on some days.

Unfortunately, the things that you do during the course of your regular day won't count towards this recommended exercise plan. Things like golf, bowling, gardening and softball are all great activities; however, they all start and stop, and start and stop. You need thirty steady minutes to boost metabolism. And while some people have perfected the art of power shopping, that doesn't count either! No one shops that hard.

Activities like swimming, bicycling and even walking will accomplish the metabolic boost that you are looking for, as long as you do it fast enough. Keep in mind, your heart does not have to be racing; it definitely has to be higher than it is when at rest. One of the best ways of gauging this is that you should have some difficulty in talking while you are exercising.

A good workout will increase your metabolism for about eighteen hours. So obviously, for best results you need to exercise at least once each day. While I recommend to my patients that they raise their heart rates for thirty minutes at least once a day, for even better results, raise the heart rate for twenty minutes twice daily. Research has shown that two short bouts of exercise stimulate the metabolism more than one longer bout. As you recall, each burst of exercise increases metabolism for about eighteen hours.

When walking or running, don't worry about distance; rather, gradually increase the pace or speed at which you exercise. It is your metabolism after exercise that burns up most of the calories.

Exercise will not only make you feel better and increase your energy level, but will help tone up muscles and skin so there is less skin sagging with the fat loss.

People have asked me many times whether it is better to exercise in the morning or in the evening. My usual answer is that the best time for them to exercise is when they are more likely to get it done. After all, getting it done is more important than when. But if I could choose, I would suggest the morning. First, once it's done you don't have to worry about unexpected events causing you to run out of time, which is likely to happen at least once in a while if you regularly exercise at the end of the day. Second, morning exercise tends to increase your metabolism for the rest of the day, and it gives you more energy.

Often people ask what type of exercise is best; once again, anything that gets your heart rate up and keeps it up for thirty minutes. Though it is also good to get exercise that will give you short bursts of especially vigorous exercise interspersed with regular exercise. At first, you would start with a burst of five or ten seconds at a time, then work up to as much as thirty or forty-five seconds of intense exercise.

Again, as with all of the things we have discussed, talk with your doctor before starting any exercise program; if you feel something unusual in your body, stop exercising for a while.

THE IMPORTANCE OF WATER

Water intake is an extremely important factor in getting results with Mesotherapy, especially when treating cellulite. When your body gets plenty of water, not only does your natural thirst return, but also you will be less hungry. Your kidneys will function better at removing waste products, reducing the load on your liver. If your liver is doing the kidneys' job of detoxifying, then it can't work as well in its task of metabolizing fat into fuel.

A person of average weight requires a minimum sixty-four ounces of water on a daily basis. Overweight people need more water because they have a larger metabolic load. The overweight person needs an additional glass of water for every twenty-five pounds of excess weight they carry around. The amount of water should also be increased to accommodate for sweating (from exercise or hot weather).

When a person's body doesn't get enough water, it begins to hold on to every drop it can. Water is stored in extra cellular spaces. The overweight person may end up with swollen hands, feet and legs, making cellulite look even worse.

Diuretics can sometimes worsen a situation. The best answer is to make sure you get plenty of water and avoid salt. You may notice that sodas can also cause water retention.

As water helps to prevent sagging skin that often accompanies weight loss, the shrinking cells are buoyed by water, which plumps the skin and leaves it healthy and vital.

CHAPTER XV

True Stories

Here are the experiences of several of my patients so you will have a better idea of how Mesotherapy progresses. Some of these I documented and others the patients wrote in their own words, telling their personal journeys with Mesotherapy. Names have been changed to protect their privacy.

ANN

A 42-year-old, white female was first seen in my office desiring Mesotherapy for upper thighs and lower abdomen. She had a history that almost caused me not to treat her. She stated that the Hashimotos Thyroiditis and lupus were under control. Fibromyositis and a history of taking steroids caused damage to her hips and both were replaced. The hip replacements were later recalled because of the silicone lubricant, and both hips were replaced again. The right hip surgery left a deep scar that looked like the Grand Canyon.

I explained to her that with her history I couldn't say she would have no problem with our treatments. Since she might have a problem with her illnesses anyway, we wouldn't know the true source of any complication.

I recommended she discuss it with her personal physician and she said she already had. She decided she was willing to accept any risk and felt comfortable with Mesotherapy. I'll have to admit, I was very hesitant. But I also felt sorry for her and really wanted to help her if I could. Since the medicine I would be using is a natural substance in her body anyway, I didn't worry so much about a problem with that. I worried more about her developing a problem unrelated to the treatments and blaming Mesotherapy. Obviously, I didn't want to go to court for malpractice, but this nice lady was probably going to have medical problems throughout her life.

What led me to go ahead and treat her were my desire to help her and the fact that she didn't seem like the type who would take advantage.

She asked me to do Mesotherapy on both upper thighs and her lower abdomen. She also asked if I could do a "touch up" around the scar area on her right leg where the fat "pooched out" around it. I told her we could probably help it some, but I couldn't make any promises.

After just one treatment, she was pleased with the results and wanted to be sure that we kept working on the scar area. After two treatments, we had the area anterior to the scar almost level with the scar, giving the appearance of a smooth surface. The area posterior to the scar was better, but still was somewhat elevated.

After the third treatment, the area around the scar was almost level with just the lowest part of the posterior area being elevated. After the fourth treatment, there were no longer any signs of the Grand Canyon and she was very pleased with the results. She was happy with the results on her thighs and abdomen also. She lost two inches in each thigh and the skin showed much better tone. And, she lost two inches in her lower abdomen.

MONETTE

"My name is Monette and I started Mesotherapy treatments to the abdomen area in mid-December 2003. I had two C-section births and I just could not get rid of the fat above the incision area. After my first treatment I lost 2½ inches in my waist! After my second treatment I could visibly see the results when looking in the mirror. I got to wear jeans that I could not fit into previously. So far, it has been two months and I have received five treatments.

"I have been dieting along with the Mesotherapy treatments and have gone from 145 pounds to 130 pounds. My waist has gone from 30 inches to 25 inches!

"As for the fat above the incision area, it is almost completely gone, and with a couple of more treatments I feel it will be gone for good!

"Because of my pregnancies I got stretch marks that were very noticeable all over my abdomen. They would not seem to fade. Now my stretch marks have faded and by just looking at them, some seem to have gone away!

"Overall, I am more than happy with the results of Mesotherapy and feel it is a safe and effective treatment for spot fat reduction."

JUDY

Judy was a highly successful businesswoman in her 40s who had liposuction in the past and was certain she never wanted to undergo that procedure again. She said, "I was down for two weeks and I still have some areas that don't look right."

She liked the idea of being able to get a treatment and then going about her business the same day without anyone knowing she even had a treatment.

She wanted to get the fat off her arms and belly. She also wanted to smooth out the "dents" in her buttocks.

We began treatment and she was doing very well in the abdomen, and the "rear" was gradually looking better. But I'm not sure she could sense the improvement in her arms. When I pinched up the arms, there was less and less fat each time, but when we measured her arms we couldn't see much change because the skin had not shrunk. Her right arm had measured larger than the left from the beginning, and she decided to stop treating the left arm but continue on the right side to see if the two sides would even out eventually. She continued treatments on the buttocks and other smaller areas we had been treating when she decided to start treatments on her double chin.

Each of the next two sessions showed good improvement, but she said that her left arm was still getting smaller. I explained to her that part of that was some of the medicine still working, and the other part of that equation was that her skin was finally getting tighter. The measurements in her arms continued to improve for over a month as the skin gradually tightened, almost like balloons after the air is let out. We just took the fat out and needed time for the skin to adjust. I explain to all of my patients that I cannot promise the skin will shrink all the way back. It depends a lot on their health and age, but most of the time the skin cooperates.

This patient has been one of my best. We have done fat and cellulite treatments just about all over her from the chin to the knees.

One day I asked her what her husband thought and she said, "I haven't told him. He just thinks I'm dieting and exercising."

I asked her how she explains the occasional bruise, and she said that with the supplements I recommended to her to prevent bruising, she hardly ever had any. But one time when he asked about a bruise, she said she just bumped into something.

KATHLEEN

"My name is Kathleen, and I am 58 years old. I began Mesotherapy spot fat reduction treatments on my stomach. I have now had six treatments and I am happy to report that I have lost 10 pounds. But more importantly, 7 inches from my waist and abdomen.

"My abdomen area has been a problem for me since the birth of my last child over twenty-four years ago. She was delivered via C-section and my stomach has never been the same. I have dieted and exercised for years trying to get these same results. I would firm up and lose weight, everywhere but there. I would always still have that "problem area" that nothing else I did could touch, until this spot fat reduction! Because of my Mesotherapy treatments, I am now able to wear my clothes without that "pooch" that used to make me so self-conscious.

"Needless to say, I am so pleased that there was help for me without having to have an invasive or dangerous surgery."

JACKIE

"May 4. I went in for my first Mesotherapy treatment with Dr. Parker today. The procedure was very quick. I think that I spent about 30 minutes in the room getting the treatment. I was expecting the shots to hurt quite a bit. The needle was pretty small though, so it didn't hurt as much as I thought that it would. I got so many shots — more than I thought that I would.

"May 11. I was a little disappointed with my results today. I only lost 1½ inches. The nurses and the doctor assured me that the results were typical and that I would get more results as the treatments went on. Those encouragements made me feel better.

"I started doing 100 sit-ups twice a day. I have been eating a low carbohydrate diet for the past year-and-a-half and have lost over 40 pounds, but I still have some fat on my tummy that I want to get rid of. I wear about a size 12 right now. I can wear some size 10s, but not often. I am getting the Mesotherapy treatments right in my abdomen.

"May 18. I knew that when I went in today that I would have great results, and I did. I lost 2 inches altogether. I could tell this week as I was putting my clothes on; my pants were looser, and other people were beginning to comment that I looked like I was losing more weight. The funny thing is that I am not really losing that much weight. I want to lose about 20 more pounds, but if I stay the same weight AND look better because of the inches that I am losing, I am happy with that.

"May 25. I am going to the gym about six times a week and loving the results that I am getting. I have lost 2½ inches specifically in the area that I wanted to target. I had been working out for months before this but had never experienced this kind of success before — WOW! I bought a size 8 pants — they are a little snug, but I bought them purposefully because I know that I am going to be able to wear them comfortably very soon. I have not worn a size 8 since before my children were born over nine years ago. After getting pregnant and having two children, I have not been able to get my body back into its former shape.

"June 8. My life got hectic after my last treatment, but I still tried to maintain healthy eating and exercising habits. With school ending, it was a little harder to get to the gym like I wanted to, but I still had success in losing inches. My total inches lost were 2. The shots hurt a little more this time than I remember in the past. The nurse encouraged me to drink a glass of water before coming in, to hydrate my body.

"June 22. This was my last treatment. I am very happy with the results today. The doctor said that he was having a hard time finding fat to inject — amazing. I know that I still have some fat to work on, but overall, the results have been great. There is no way that I could have lost this much in this little time on my own.

"July 6. My final measurements were taken today. I lost a total of 12 inches and 6 inches in the area around my waist, which is the area of my body that I hated the most. I feel so much better about looking at myself in the mirror. I don't have to suck in my tummy when I am putting on my size 8 pants. In fact, I have had to buy quite a few new clothes (size 8 and even a few 6s!) that will fit me now. I think that I am looking better than I did even before I had kids! My tummy is flatter, and I definitely feel better about how I look than I ever have before."

SALLY

Sally and her mother, both beautiful women, came to get Mesotherapy treatments. Since both were attractive and trim, I wasn't sure how they thought I could improve on what God had already given them. But, bless their hearts, they wanted to look even better.

I was surprised when Sally slipped off her jeans to show me her legs, her main area of concern. She really did have reason for alarm. A lot of cellulite, and she was very embarrassed by it. Sally was engaged to be married and wanted to look amazing before her honeymoon.

Sally responded extremely well to the treatments. She

lost inches as well as cellulite. As is often the case, I had to begin using less medicine for fat removal and more medicine for cellulite reduction. As the treatments progressed, it was harder to find any fat.

I almost hated to see those two women respond so quickly. They had such wonderful personalities and were a lot of fun to be around. My staff also hated to see them go.

EMILY

"My name is Emily and this is my Mesotherapy story. I have three children, and as each child was born I noticed my 'baby pooch' increasing.

"I had used Dr. Parker's diet programs after having my children to lose the baby weight and they worked great. I just seemed to have the one area in my lower abdomen that I couldn't get rid of.

"I started Mesotherapy, very skeptically, in November. After my first week of treatment in my abdomen area, I lost a total of 2½ inches. I was so amazed and pleased.

"After two weeks of treatment I had lost enough that Dr. Parker was able use the same amount of treatment and start working on my 'love handles.'

"After four total treatments I was thrilled! I felt comfortable in my body again. I felt and looked like I had prior to having children.

"It has been seven months since I took Meso treatments and I love the results. I have not gained any weight or inches back and I feel wonderful!"

AMANDA

Amanda, a 33-year-old mother of two, had tried several ways to lose weight after a C-section with her second child. She had lost weight, but was still struggling with fat that had pocketed by her scar from the C-section.

"I have tried exercise and dieted, and I did lose weight, but there are just those areas that aren't going away," she said. She visited with me in May 2004, and decided to try Mesotherapy for her abdominal area.

About eight weeks later, after six treatments, the measurement around Amanda's waist at her bellybutton had gone from 35½ inches to 29¾ inches.

"I've tried lots of things to target my areas of fat that were hanging on after all those years. I've tried hard to get rid of them. Mesotherapy is wonderful; it's the best thing I could have done. It got me off that plateau."

TONYA

A 42-year-old woman came into my office wanting Mesotherapy treatment for cellulite in her legs.

"It's really bad when your teenage daughter tells you that you need to do something," she stated.

I explained to her that cellulite goes a little slower than spot fat reduction, and that she may need as many as ten or twelve sessions to get the results she was hoping for. I was sure we could help her, but I couldn't make any promises, as everybody is different.

After her second treatment, I asked her if she had told her daughter what she was doing.

She said, "NO, I'm just going to wait and see if she notices." She said that her daughter was away at her grandparents' and she would just wait and see how things went when her daughter got home.

When this patient came in for her fourth treatment, she was ecstatic.

"I'm so pleased. I picked my daughter up at the airport and she asked me if I'd lost weight. She said, 'Your legs look better.' I kept asking her if she really thought so, because I loved hearing it."

I asked her if she told her daughter what she was doing. She said, "No, I still haven't told her anything."

But I'm sure she will eventually! And, probably other people, too.

KEITH

Keith, a musician, was concerned about looking his best because he was preparing to shoot his first music video. He wanted to fix his double chin and improve his abdominal area. He told me he wanted his abs to look "ripped." He was a giant of a man — looked like he could play for the Dallas Cowboys.

He followed the program exceptionally well. His double chin improved dramatically with just two treatments. After just four treatments he had lost four inches in his waist and was on his way to developing those "ripped" abs he was looking for.

He said he had friends who played for the Dallas Cowboys and he once went with them to a practice. Some of the practice squad players thought he was a new player and one of them was going to be cut.

Keith was nice enough to agree to be my model for a training session. I had a group of physicians in town one weekend for training and I was able to use him to demonstrate the double chin treatment.

I remember how he raved about how great he was doing and how Mesotherapy was helping him. I was disappointed that I did not have my tape recorder running at the time. Fortunately, one of the other physicians had her recorder on and promised to make me a copy. He unknowingly, and completely uncoerced, gave me enough sound bites to make commercials for the next several years.

These are just a few examples of our Mesotherapy successes. I have many more. Some people will do better than others. All I can do is the analysis and injections. The rest is up to the individual to eat right and exercise properly. If they do that, they will usually be successful in getting the results they desire in those hard-to-get areas.

CHAPTER XVI

Mesotherapy Do's and Don'ts

1. For twenty-four hours following Mesotherapy you must avoid the following:
   a. Massaging or rubbing the area
   b. Bathing or swimming (You may shower, but you may not use soap.)
   c. Soap, cream or lotions to the area
   d. Sun exposure to the treated area
2. The following supplements will enhance results:
   a. EPA helps lower triglycerides released by the therapy
   b. L-Carnitine
   c. Master Fiber detoxifies colon and liver
   d. Green Tea, especially when taken right before exercise
3. Exercise:
   a. Cardiovascular for thirty minutes, three times a week
   b. Muscle toning for thirty minutes, three times a week
4. The following injections will enhance results:
   a. AMP increases natural metabolism
   b. Lipotropic helps liver to process and remove fat
5. Results will be better if you avoid:
   a. Starches

b. Sugar

c. Trans fats (margarine, fried foods, chips, etc.)

6. For special occasions, we recommend:
    a. Absorba-fat, which blocks fat absorption
    b. Carb-blaster blocks absorption of carbohydrate calories

7. To return skin elasticity, firmness, and reduce stretch marks:
    a. Vita Crème contains CoQ10 — lightens, brightens, and tightens skin. The ultimate "wrinkle cure," Vita Crème increases moisture by up to 40 percent.
    b. Or try Derma Q-gel, also with a high concentration of CoQ10 — efficient antioxidant and moisturizer that reduces inflammation.
    c. Drink eight 8-oz. glasses of water daily

CHAPTER XVII

Cellulite Protocol

Mix 4 ounces unsweetened cranberry or grape juice with 28 ounces of water. Drink a half-gallon per day.
1-2 Lipotropic shots per week
2 Master Fiber capsules per day
2-6 EPA capsules per day
1-3 GLA capsules per day
3 CLA capsules per day (a.m.) — with guarana, which stimulates metabolism
1-2 teaspoons flaxseed oil per day
1 Rodex Forte capsule per day
1 Prevenzyme capsule three times a day on an empty stomach
Avoid salt, soda, sugar, starches, trans and saturated fats

CHAPTER XVIII

How to Choose a Mesotherapist

In Appendix 1 is a list of physicians who practice Mesotherapy. This is by no means a complete list. There are more physicians being trained all the time. Just because a physician is on this list does not guarantee that he/she is the most qualified physician in your area to perform Mesotherapy. I do think you will find that most of these physicians are very qualified.

It is up to you to do your homework. Ask them where they were trained and how much training they have had. Some physicians may attend a talk on Mesotherapy and say they know everything they need to know. That is not good enough! But they do not need to have as much training as I have had. I wanted to receive as much training as I could, and by different physicians from around the world. This way, I would be able to do the best possible job for my patients. I could also do a better job of teaching the many physicians I have trained from all over the country.

Ask the physician where they received training and if they have a certificate. Ask how long they have been doing Mesotherapy and if they belong to a Mesotherapy association.

Of course, one of the best ways to know if a physician is for you is to visit with them personally. See if you feel comfortable with the facility, the staff, and especially with the physician.

Last but not least, ask for recommendations from other people.

Again, the list is just to help you get started in finding a Mesotherapist. Be sure to do your own research.

CHAPTER XIX

Transdermal Application — the Future of Mesotherapy

While applying my transdermal (absorbed through the skin) testosterone cream one day, I thought to myself, "There must be a way to apply special ingredients in this same manner that would help in fat metabolism. What a unique way to help my patients get results." Obviously they could observe positive effects all over because it would be absorbed and transported to other areas of the body also, but it would be especially effective at the site of application.

The next questions were, "Could I develop a formula of natural substances similar to what we use in Mesotherapy injections? Could I find someone that could develop a similar delivery system to what I used to replace my testosterone?" I knew that many medications were being developed employing transdermal patches and creams, so the possibility was certainly there.

Shortly thereafter, I was giving a seminar on Mesotherapy in Phoenix. I began to visit with a friend of mine, who happens to own a pharmaceutical company. When I brought up my idea about this new topical form of Mesotherapy, he said he had just recently developed a unique system that could do just what I was thinking of, and he had a patent on it. I told him what formula would be necessary for it to be effective, and he said he would see what he could do.

Just a few short months later, he had it, and it was ready for me to try. He thought it was a winner. He had added a few other ingredients to make it work better on the skin. He asked me to look it over, and if I liked it, he could put it in an applicator bottle that would dispense even doses every time.

After a few weeks of going back and forth with discussions on the final product, we realized we hadn't given it a name. We finally agreed on *MesoDerm*. I asked him to manufacture a batch and I would test it on myself, and if I liked it I would ask some patients to give it a try. We would do a clinical trial right here in my office. I tried it on a group of six patients. Five of them loved the new product. The sixth did not, and stopped using the *MesoDerm* altogether. All six patients were on my regular weight loss program and following an exercise program as suggested. All six lost weight and inches. But the five who had used the cream had noticeably greater results. Needless to say, the sixth patient is back using the cream and much happier.

I was then asked by another company, Nuvo Concepts, if they could make our cream and market it nationally. Since I am one of their medical advisors, I directed them to my friend at the pharmaceutical company. My friend had been marketing *MesoDerm* to physicians, and I thought the two companies might be able to come to an agreement that would satisfy everyone involved. They came to such an agreement and are planning to market the product under the name *Mesunique.*

They have tested it on more patients, and the results have been very impressive. *Patients are saying that they can see changes in the skin tone in as early as two weeks.*

Mesunique is ideal for people who cannot find a Meso-therapy specialist near them or cannot afford Mesotherapy injections or are simply afraid of needles. All of these people can now experience the same amazing results as Meso-therapy treatments. I believe that this transdermal application will be the future of Mesotherapy. In fact, I am now encouraging my patients to take this less expensive, safer, and less painful route even though it is not as financially beneficial for me. I just believe it is that much better.

Remember, just like with the Mesotherapy injections, we are just *helping*. You are the one that makes it work by eating right, avoiding the bad fats, exercising right, and taking supplements that help support the liver and increase your metabolism safely.

Along these lines, I have also developed a new formulation for Nuvo Concepts to go with *Mesunique*; this product is called *Accelerator*.

The *Accelerator* contains ingredients that will help curb appetite, decrease sugar and starch cravings, and improve fat metabolism. The *Accelerator* makes the program safe and easy to do yourself. Used in conjunction with *Mesunique*, a sensible diet and exercise, our patients are getting tremendous results.

Now I feel we can finally reverse the statistics showing that over 60 percent of the people in the U.S. are overweight. Using all of these tools I have mentioned here, I believe everyone can now be on the road to the good health and the good figures we all desire.

THE ACCELERATOR FORMULA

Hydroxycitric acid: This formula contains one of the safest and most effective appetite suppressants available. It is also a well established fat burning agent. It is known to inhibit lipid synthesis and lower the formation of LDL and triglycerides.

Methionine: Considered one of the body's most powerful detoxifying agents, it helps prevent damage to the liver and acts as a lipotropic agent to help prevent excess fat build up in the liver and the body. It is a very good antioxidant.

Inositol: A nutrient that works in conjunction with methionine and choline to prevent the accumulation of fats. It also participates in the action of serotonin, a neurotransmitter known to control mood appetite.

Choline: Along with inositol it prevents fats from accumulating in the liver and facilitates metabolism and the removal of fat. It is essential for the health of the liver, increases HDL levels, and converts fats into useful products.

Chromium: This mineral is probably the most crucial nutrient involved in sugar metabolism! It is also essential for lipid metabolism. It promotes fat loss while at the same time helping to retain lean body mass (muscle). Without this nutrient, people on diets tend to lose fat *and* muscle. Chromium appears to decrease sugar and carbohydrate cravings, normalize sugar levels, raise good cholesterol (HDL), and lower bad cholesterol LDL and triglycerides.

Adenosine: Causes fat cells to release their stored fat so it can be burned as energy. This process happens in the Kreb's cycle (energy cycle). Studies show that in most overweight people, there is not enough AMP in this cycle to initiate fat burning. Adenosine changes that, and the increased fat burning improves overall energy levels naturally without the nervous side effects that are seen with most stimulants.

Physicians can obtain the *MesoDerm* cream and most of the products I have mentioned here from Legere Pharmaceuticals. Physicians can contact Legere at 1-800-528-3144.

Consumers can obtain ***Mesunique***, the ***Accelerator*** and most of the other products from Nuvo Concepts at www.nuvoconcepts.com and www.mesunique.com.

CHAPTER XX

Summary

In these pages, I have shown you a good deal of information about Mesotherapy — its development, how it works, what is used in treatments, and what you can expect from them. We have reviewed some of the FAQ's and shown you results of tests and studies so you now know that this procedure is extremely safe and effective when done by a qualified, well-trained physician.

I am sure you understand by now that the final results depend on you as much as the physician. It takes both of you doing your jobs to get the desired results.

Hopefully, you now have an understanding of fat metabolism, and sugars and starches, and how they have definite effects on the results.

I have given you some exercise ideas that I trust will get you started on your own regimen. These will make the results even better.

From here, it is up to you to find a Mesotherapist that you feel comfortable with, and then follow the program to see what wonderful results you can obtain. I expect you will do as well as most of my patients.

Hopefully in Appendix 1 you will find a Mesotherapist who you will be happy with. And in Appendix 2, find sources for all the supplements you need.

Good luck and God bless!

Appendix 1

Qualified Mesotherapists
(Listed by State)

Dr. Suneil Jain 8390 E. Via de Ventura, Suite F-111, Scottsdale, AZ 85258 (480) 951-6506

Denette King, N.M.D. 2127 E. Baseline Rd., Suite 103, Tempe, AZ 85283 (602) 750-5039

Mariam Malek, N.D. 7200 W. Bell Rd., Scottsdale, AZ 85255

J. D. McCoy, N.M.D. 3111 W. Chandler Blvd., Suite 1104, Chandler, AZ 85226 (480) 855-7546

Grant McKernan, N.M.D. 10177 N. 92nd St., Suite 102, Scottsdale, AZ 85258 (480) 860-0300

Patrick Mulcahy, D.O. 410 N. Malacate St., Ajo, AZ 85321 (520) 387-5706

Glen Ozalan, N.M.D. 1107 E. Bell Rd., Phoenix, AZ 85022 (602) 866-3500

Stacey Raybuck, D.O. 10340 N. 117th Pl., Scottsdale, AZ 85259 (480) 556-1833

Bradley Smith, N.M.D. 1050 E. Southern, Suite 4, Tempe, AZ 85282 (480) 343-1576

James Tuggle, N.M.D. 8880 E. Via Linda, Suite 107, Scottsdale, AZ 85258 (480) 314-0388

James Yarruso, M.D. 10950 N. LaCanada, #9101, Tucson, AZ 85737 (520) 544-0477

ARKANSAS

Greg Pineau, D.O. 636 West Broadway, North Little Rock, AR (501) 374-6213

CALIFORNIA

William S. Anapoell, M.D. 4060 Fourth Ave., Suite 508, San Diego, CA 92103 (619) 987-2713

Sam Assassa, M.D. 9135 W. Olympic Blvd., Beverly Hills, CA 90212 (310) 247-0633

Gerald Bock, M.D. 1502 St Marks Plaza, #8, #9, Stockton, CA 95207 (209) 957-0720

Emmanuel Brandeis, M.D. 239 S. LaCienega Blvd., Suite 101, Beverly Hills, CA 90211 (310) 855-7504

Daniel B. Brubaker, D.O. 3726 N. First St., Fresno, CA 93726 (559) 248-0116

Steven Burres, M.D. 465 N. Raybury Dr., Suite 1012, Beverly Hills, CA 90210 (310) 385-0590

Robert H. Cohen, M.D. 7901 Santa Monica Blvd., Suite 101, West Hollywood, CA 90046 (213) 400-8875

Glenn A. Cooperman, M.D. 8380 Morro Rd., Atascadero, CA 93422 (805) 466-7773

Frances Dee Filgas, M.D. 24204 Geyserville Ave., Cloverdale, CA 95425 (707) 857-4182

Gwen Flagg, M.D. 16812 S. Hawthorne Blvd., Lawndale, CA 90260 (310) 371-1100

William L. Heimer II, M.D. 320 Santa Fe Drive, #310, Encinitas, CA 92024 (760) 944-7000

Peter Helton, M.D. 2011 Westcliff Dr., Suite 9, Newport Beach, CA 92660 (949) 646-3376

Sid Kamrava, M.D. 18411 Clark St., Suite 301, Tarzana, CA 91356 (818) 705-0032

Jane F. Kardashian, M.D. 6769 N. Fresno St., Fresno, CA 93710 (559) 435-0337

Marketa Limova, M.D. 1340 W. Herndon Ave., Suite 101, Fresno, CA 93711 (559) 438-6577

Victor Liu, M.D. 1720 El Camino Real, Suite 200, Burlingame, CA 94010

Evelyne Llorente, M.D. 11180 Warner Ave., Suite 257, Fountain Valley, CA 92708 (714) 885-8980

Joel Lopez, M.D. 345 N. Portal Ave., 2nd Floor, San Francisco, CA 94217 (415) 566-1000

Denise R. Mark, M.D. 659 Abrego St., Suite 6, Monterey, CA 93940 (831) 642-9266

Gustavo Marks, M.D. 22201 Sherman Way, Canoga Park, CA 91303 (818) 999-5900

Gilbert Martinez, M.D. 12598 Central Ave., Chino, CA 91710 (909) 627-3300

Faye Montegrande, M.D. 321 N. Larchmont Blvd. #824, Los Angeles, CA 90004 (323) 464-0286

Raphael Nach, M.D. 435 N. Roxbury Dr. #207, Beverly Hills, CA 90210 (310) 858-4493

Kendrick Ng, M.D. 903 Berkebile Ct., Monterey Park, CA 91755 (626) 665-2814

Byung-Ho Pak, M.D. 9012 Garden Grove Blvd. #1, Garden Grove, CA 92844 (714) 539-7700

Samuel Perez, M.D. 45541 Oasis St., Indio, CA 92201 (760) 347-3113

Bipin Patel, M.D. 9508 Stockdale Highway, Suite 140, Bakersfield, CA 93331 (661) 847-7546

Pravin Patel, M.D. 1190 E. Paseo El Mirador, Palm Springs, CA 92262 (760) 864-9993

Andrea Cole Raub, D.O. 12264 El Camino Real, Suite 204, San Diego, CA 92130 (858) 724-1313

Roy Robinson, M.D. 10159 Mission George Rd. #A, Santee, CA 92071 (858) 288-6056

Adam Rotunda, M.D. UCLA, Box 956957, 200 Medical Plaza, Suite 45, Los Angeles, CA 90095

Michael Schorr, M.D. 2001 E. Orangeberg, Modesto, CA 95555

Bharati Shah, M.D. 22909 Lazy Trail, Diamond Bar, CA 91765 (714) 932-7593

George Sun, M.D. 624 West Juarte Rd. #102, Arketa, CA 91007 (626) 447-0118

I-Wen Tseng, D.O. 2204 Q Street, Suite A, Bakersfield, CA 93301 (661) 321-0988

Gregory G. Williams, M.D. 2205 19th St., Bakersfield, CA 93301 (661) 324-8346

Celedonia Yue, M.D. 6673 Foothill Blvd., Tujunga, CA 91042 (818) 353-8581

Edwin Yuen, M.D. 760 Market St., Suite 408, San Francisco, CA 94102 (415) 296-7777

Filiberto Zadini, M.D. 7012 Reseda Blvd., Suite A, Reseda, CA 91335 1-877-MESO-MED

Giorgio Zadini, M.D. 7012 Reseda Blvd., Suite A, Reseda, CA 91335 1-877-MESO-MED

COLORADO

Kenneth G. Oleszek, M.D. 3234 W. 23rd Ave., Denver, CO 80211 (720) 628-8570

Alexis Parker, M.D. 760 South Colorado Blvd., Suite M, Denver, CO 80246 (303) 782-5082

CONNECTICUT

Sharon Juliet Littzi, M.D. 1 Morse Court, New Canaan, CT 06840 (203) 966-2336

FLORIDA

Allyn A. Brizel, M.D. 4800 North Federal Highway, Suite C, Boca Raton, FL 33431 (561) 367-9101

Robert Brueck, M.D. 3700 Central Ave., Fort Myers, FL 33901 (239) 939-5233

Luis Cruz, M.D. 3233 Palm Ave., Hialeah, FL 33012 (786) 277-6915

Jay Garcia, M.D. 13905 Carrollwood Village Run, Tampa, FL 33618

Enrique Gomez, M.D. 3233 Palm Ave., Hialeah, FL 33012

Jeffrey Hunt, D.O. 3001 N. Rocky Point Dr., Suite 125, Tampa, FL 33607 1-800-499-8346

Abdala Kalil, M.D. 844 Alton Rd., 2nd Floor, Miami Beach, FL 33139 1-866-352-6869

Manuel Martinez 10031 SW 40th St., Miami, FL 33165 (305) 225-7546

Jacqueline Redondo, M.D. 10300 Sunset Dr., Suite 282, Miami, FL 33173 (305) 412-2800

Paul Rose, M.D. 120 S. Fremont, Tampa, FL 33606

Daniel Stein, M.D. 2815 W. Virginia Ave., Suite A, Tampa, FL 33607 1-888-973-3832

GEORGIA

Truett Bridges, M.D. 4920 Roswell Rd., Suite 35, Atlanta, GA 30342 (404) 843-8880

Marcia V. Byrd, M.D. 11050 Crabapple Rd., Bldg. B, Suite 105, Roswell, GA 30075 (770) 587-1711

Jean L. Chapman, M.D. 3005 Old Alabama Rd., Alpharetta, GA 30022 (678) 990-4900

Kendra Cole, M.D. 3655 Howell Ferry Rd., Suite 400, Duluth, GA 30096 (678) 417-6900

Nancy Ellwood, M.D. 1811 Edwina Dr., Vidalia, GA 30474 (912) 537-9779

Jim Lingle, M.D. 455 E. Paces Ferry Rd. NE, Suite 205, Atlanta, GA 30305 (404) 264-0800

Joyce Poag, M.D. P.O. Box 1119, Suwanee, GA 30024

Ava Bell-Taylor, M.D. 1150 Hammon Dr. NE, Bldg. D, Suite 4230, Atlanta, GA 30328 (708) 848-7763

HAWAII

Choon Kia Yeo, M.D. 1650 Liliha St., Suite 102, Honolulu, HI 96817 (808) 528-0888

ILLINOIS

Georgia A. Davis, M.D. 1112 Rickard Rd., Suite B, Springfield, IL 62704 (217) 787-9540

Marsha E. Gorens, M.D. 6342 S. Polasky Rd., Chicago 60629 (773) 284-8601

Ross A. Hauser, M.D. 715 Lake St., Suite 600, Oak Park, IL 60301 (708) 848-7789

Joseph Z. Hura, M.D. 22 W. Calendar Ave., Suite E, LaGrange, IL 60525 (708) 354-3000

Marc S. Karlan, M.D. 201 E. Huron St., Suite 10-100, Chicago, IL 60611 (312) 944-2424

Monte J. Meldman, M.D. 3833 S. Mission Hills Rd., Northbrook, IL 60062 (847) 236-9999

William R. Panje, M.D. 999 N. Lake Shore Dr., 4th Floor, Chicago, IL 60611 (309) 663-8311

John L. Poag II, M.D. 1401 Eastland Dr., Bloomingdale, IL 61701 (309) 661-3324

Razvan Rentea, M.D. 6167 Caldwell, Chicago, IL 60646 (773) 583-7793

INDIANA

Larry W. Banyash, M.D. 23631 US 33 S., Suite A, Elkhart, IN 46517 (574) 875-1146

Leonard Dale Guyer, M.D. 836 E. 86 St., Indianapolis, IN 86240 (317) 580-9355

Joseph P. Bark, M.D. 1401 Harrodsburg Rd., Lexington, KY 40504

James Cunningham, M.D. 2500 Richmond, Box 216, Mt. Vernon, KY 40456 (606) 256-4102

Lena D. Edwards, M.D. 1001 Monarch St., Suite 110, Lexington, KY 40513 (859) 224-3026

Susan E. Neil, M.D. 2101 Nicholasville Rd., Suite 206, Lexington, KY 40503 (859) 278-6345

LOUISIANA

Robert Fortier-Bensen, M.D. 723 N. Causeway Blvd., Mandeville, LA 70448 (985) 630-5196

MARYLAND

John K. Aziz, M.D. 5452 Ring Dove Lane, Columbia, MD 21044

Doriscine Colley, M.D. 9020 Bruno Road, Randallstown, MD 21133 (410) 521-0848

MASSACHUSETTS

Sandra V. Kristiansen, M.D. 176 East Main St., Suite 4, Westborough, MA 01581 (508) 870-5900

Elliot Lach, M.D. 77 Turnpike Rd., Southboro, MA 01772 (508) 481-0300

MICHIGAN

Manuel E. Garcia, M.D. 4121 Okemos Rd., Suite 23, Okemos, MI 48864 (517) 381-0000

Robert Grafton, M.D. 555 Barclay Circle, Suite 140, Rochester Hills, MI 48307 (248) 299-6228

Robert Lamberts, M.D. 655 Kenmoor SE, Grand Rapids, MI 49546 (616) 949-5600

Charles Mok, D.O. 8180 26 Mile Road, Suite 105, Shelby Township, MI 48316 1-800-593-5136

Robert G. Saieg, M.D. 44199 Dequindre Road, Suite 408, Troy, MI 48085 (248) 828-8484

MINNESOTA

Harold Seim, M.D. 180 Liberty Parkway, Stillwater, MN 55082 (803) 796-3820

MISSOURI

Richard Bligh, M.D. 777 S. New Ballas, Suite 200, East St. Louis, MO 63141 (314) 994-1536

Edward McDonagh, D.O. 2800-A Kendallwood Pkwy., Kansas City, MO 64119 (816) 453-5940

Kenneth Rotskoff, M.D. 260 Prince Towne Dr., St. Louis, MO 63141 (314) 576-6659

NEVADA

Joan S. Leks, M.D. 7272 Palmyra Ave., Las Vegas, NV 88117 (702) 630-1854

Murray M. Rosenberg, M.D. 2931 N. Tenaya Way, Suite 106, Las Vegas, NV 89128 (702) 838-0400

NEW JERSEY

Todd F. Boff, M.D. 282 South Ave., Fanwood, NJ 07023 (908) 889-4600

Cheryl S. Citron, M.D. 315 E. Northfield Rd. 2A, Livingston, NJ 07039 (973) 535-3200

Joseph A. De Marco, Jr. 24 Godwin Ave., 2nd Floor, Midland Park, NJ 07432 (201) 447-1160

Allan Magaziner, D.O. 1151 Barbara Drive, Cherry Hill, NJ 08003 (856) 424-8222

Marco Pelosi, M.D. 350 Kennedy Blvd., Bayonne, NJ 07002 (201) 858-1800

Neil L. Rosen, D.O. 555 Shrewsbury Ave., Shrewsbury, NJ 07702 (732) 219-0894

Robert Sawicki, D.O. 1 Distribution Way, Monmouth Junction, NJ 08852 (908) 925-2422

Steven Streit, M.D. 4710 US Highway 9, Howell, NJ 07731 (732) 367-5330

Susan Stevens Tanne, M.D. 290 South Livingston Ave., 1st Floor, Livingston, NJ 07039 1-800-618-6376

NEW MEXICO

Robert Dean Blair, D.O. 101 Hospital Loop NE, Suite 209, Albuquerque, NM 87105 (505) 881-1532

Wolfgang Haese, M.D. 2465 Bataan Memorial West, Suite 2, Las Cruces, NM 88012 (505) 373-8415

Ralph J. Luciani, D.O., M.D. 10601 Lomas Blvd. NE, Suite 103, Albuquerque, NM 87112 (505) 298-5995

NEW YORK

Lance I. Austein, M.D. 1913 Avenue Z, Brooklyn, NY 11235 (718) 934-6661

Michael Belfiore, D.O. 275 Rockaway Turnpike, Lawrence, NY 11559 (516) 371-5800

Alexander J. Covey, M.D. 445 Main St., Center Moriches, NY 11934 (631) 878-9200

Oleg Davie, M.D. 133-A West End Ave., Brooklyn, NY 11235 (718) 743-5616

Eric Dohner, M.D. 70 Delaware St., Walton, NY 13856 (607) 865-5800

Zhanna Kanevsky, M.D. 1763 E. 12th St, Brooklyn, NY 11229 (718) 376-7766

Michael Kaplan, D.O. 325 Middle Country Rd., Smithtown, NY 11787 (631) 366-2331

Alexander Kulick, M.D. 625 Madison Ave., New York, NY 10022 (212) 838-8265

Everett Lautin, M.D. 885 Park Ave., New York, NY 10021 (212) 535-0229

Shirley Madhere, M.D. 430 West Broadway, 2nd Floor, New York, NY 10012 (212) 941-1571

Dr. Shahid Rasul 5143 Bell Blvd., Bayside, NY 11364 (917) 774-1787

Steve Salvatore, M.D. 111 E. 88th St. Apt. 7A, New York, NY 10128 (212) 688-5882

Joseph Sciammarella, M.D. 230 Hilton Ave., Suite 230, Hempstead, NY 11550 (516) 485-6667

Jyotindra G. Shah, M.D. 20 Ilinka Lane, Irvington, NY 10533 (914) 591-6770

Halina Stec, M.D. 619 Bronx River Rd., Yonkers, NY 10704 (914) 968-7938

Roxana L. Todriascu, M.D. Astoria, NY 11103 (347) 612-2929

NORTH CAROLINA

Rashid A. Buttar, D.O. 20721 Torrence Chapel Rd., Suite 101-103, Cornelius, NC 28031 (704) 895-9355

Jose Gonzalez, M.D. 2270 Hendersonville Rd., Unit A, Arden, NC 28704 (828) 684-4462

NORTH DAKOTA

Yvonne Gomez, M.D. 205 Palin Hills Dr., Grand Forks, ND 58201 (701) 795-2240

OHIO

Navkaran Singh, M.D. 3648 Edwards Rd., Cincinnati, OH 45208 (513) 924-1200

Maria V. Soto, D.O. 4678 Maystar Way, Hillard, OH 43026 (614) 777-8060

OKLAHOMA

Joan M. Hardt, M.D. 1404 E. 9th St., Edmond, OK 73034 (405) 348-5297

Michael Steelman, M.D. 13301 N. Meridian, Bldg. 400, Oklahoma City, OK 73120 (405) 755-4837

Ray Zimmer, D.O. 602 N. Dalton, Valliant, OK 74058 (580) 933-4235

OREGON

Adam Maddox, N.D. 811 NW 19th Ave., Suite 104, Portland, OR 97209 (503) 241-3579

Sharon Stubbs, M.D. 913 NW Garden Valley Blvd., Rosebury, OR 97470-6513

Elizabeth VanderVeer, M.D. 6650 SW Redwood Lane, Suite 150, Portland, OR 97224 (503) 443-2250

Roger Erro, M.D. 551 Lon Acre Lane, Yardley, PA 19067 (215) 291-9377

Alexander S. Fine, M.D. 834 Ayrgale, Philadelphia, PA 19128 (215) 744-5505

Scott Leone, D.O. 5700 Corporate Dr., Suite 265, Pittsburgh, PA 15327 (412) 369-5900

Harvey Levin, M.D. 1709 Packer Ave., Philadelphia, PA 19145 (215) 467-0200

Kurt Moran, M.D. 600 Lackawanna Ave., Scranton, PA 18503 (570) 963-0766

RHODE ISLAND

Dariusz Nasiek, M.D. 225 Vaucluse Ave., Middletown, RI 02842 (401) 388-8666

SOUTH CAROLINA

Pierre Jaffe, M.D. One Medical Plaza, Suite 240, Columbia, SC 29203 (803) 256-6648

Adrienne Labotka, M.D. 500 Squire's Pointe, Suite B, Duncan, SC 29334 (864) 433-8980

Ben M. Treen, M.D. 9 Hawthorne Rd., Greenville, SC 29615 (864) 288-7171

TENNESSEE

John Binhlam, M.D. 10 Cadillac Dr., Suite 120, Brentwood, TN 37027 (615) 843-7546

Connie L. Catron, M.D. 49 Cleveland St., Suite 320, Crossville, TN 38555 (931) 456-5331

Richard B. Gibbs, M.D. 1215 Poplar Ave., Memphis, TN 38104 (901) 274-8668

H. Joseph Holliday, M.D. 1005 W. Madison Ave., Athens, TN 37303 (423) 744-7540

Phillip Langsdon, M.D. 7499 Poplar Pike, Germantown, TN 38138 (901) 755-6465

David Livingston, M.D. 1567 N. Eastman Road, Suite 4, Kingsport, TN 37664 (423) 245-667

TEXAS

Gary Albertson, D.O. 211 RR. 620 South, Suite 120, Austin, TX 78734 (512) 266-6713

G. R. Albertson, D.O. 8024 Mesa Dr., Suite 114, Austin, TX 79756 (915) 943-9477

Sylvan Bartlett, M.D. 750 W. 5th St., Odessa, TX 79761 (432) 585-5777

Alberto L. Belalcazar, M.D. 3242 S. Alameda, Corpus Christi, TX 78404 (361) 888-6255

Raymond Brewer, M.D. 9614 Pipe Creek St., San Antonio, TX 78251 (210) 273-1143

Manuel R. Carrasco, M.D. 801 Caprock Dr., Big Spring, TX 79720 (432) 714-4500

James Chepko, M.D. 1303 Antigua Lane, Houston, TX 77058 (713) 694-9000

Mike Clark, Natural Biohealth 211 RR. 620 South, Suite 120, Austin, TX 78734 (512) 266-6713

Arthur Hadley, M.D. 11777 Katy Freeway, Suite 270, Houston, TX 77079 (218) 597-1010

Donald L. Hall, M.D. 2901 North 10th, Suite A-B, McAllen, TX 78504

Richard Leconey, M.D. 3120 SW Freeway, Suite 400, Houston, TX 77098 (713) 807-1000

Lufkin R. Moses, D.O. 27 Club Terrace, Sweetwater, TX 79556 (325) 235-1132

Raul Najera, M.D. 7878 Gateway East #202, El Paso, TX 79915 (915) 590-1662

Sameena Rasheed, 1504 Lotus Ln., Longview, TX 75604 (903) 445-4911

Deidre Rhoads, M.D. 211 RR. 620 South, Suite 120, Austin, TX 78734 (512) 266-6713

Larry Richardson, M.D. 25000 Pitkin, Suite 120, Spring, TX 77386 (281) 367-0070

James Robles, M.D. 412 E. 18th St., Weslaco, TX 78596 (956) 447-9396

Ernest Roman, M.D. 11211 Katy Freeway, Suite 425, Houston, TX 77079 (713) 827-2220

Anna Rosinska, M.D. 713 Pinehurst Dr., Midland, TX 79705 (432) 264-1500

Kevin Smith, M.D. 6410 Fannin #810, Houston, TX 77030 (713) 795-0600

John T. Taylor, D.O. 4714 S. Western, Amarillo, TX 79109 (806) 355-8263

Carlos Toledo, M.D. 1712 Highway 3 (Old Galveston Rd.), Houston, TX 77079 (713) 923-4765

Humberto J. Varela, M.D. 506 Gale, Laredo, TX 78041 (956) 727-8760

Michael Walker, M.D. 206 W. Windcrest, Fredericksburg, TX 78624 (830) 997-0252

Lyle D. Weeks, M.D. 1700 N. Oregon, Suite 755, El Paso, TX 79902 (915) 541-1225

Michelle Zaniewski-Singh, M.D. 17070 Red Oak Dr., Suite 309, Houston, TX 77090 (281) 580-7401

Dario Zuniga, M.D. 6550 Mapleridge, Suite 122, Houston, TX 77081 (713) 665-3428

UTAH

Harry Adelson, M.D. 2188 S. Highland Dr., Suite 210, Salt Lake City, UT 84106 (810) 582-3260

Robin Berger, M.D. 640 East 700 South, Suite 2, St. George, UT 84770 (435) 673-7546

VIRGINIA

David Ali, M.D. 1825 Samuel Morse Dr., Reston, VA 20190 (730) 787-9866

Jo Bohannon, M.D. 2306 Robious Station Circle, Midlothian, VA 23113 (804) 378-3048

Denise Brunner, M.D. 5015 Lee Hwy., Suite 201, Arlington, VA 22207 (703) 558-4980

WASHINGTON

Eduardo Castro, M.D. P.O. Box 44, Troutdale, VA 24378 (276) 677-3631

Peter Cooperrider, M.D. 12911 120th Ave. NE, Kirkland, WA 98034 (425) 899-4149

Keith Levitt, M.D. 1417 4th Ave., Suite 510, Seattle, WA 98101 (206) 622-5300

Lucinda Messer, M.D. 1313 Market St., Suite 3000, Kirkland, WA 98033 (425) 827-9770

Virginia T. Stevens, M.D. 14024 NE 181st St. #201, Woodinville, WA 98027 866-424-3416

WEST VIRGINIA

Cynthia Martinsen, D.O. 1301 Elizabeth Pike, Elizabeth, WV 26143 (304) 485-2700

WISCONSIN

Manelle Fernando, 15 W. Milwaukee, Suite 206, Taresville, WI 53548 (608) 756-0791

Appendix 2

Supplements — Where to Find Them

Obviously, some of these supplements can be found at your local health food store. Most of these can be obtained at my office, but many can be purchased through the supplier below. Keep in mind, these prices are subject to change without notice.

Advanced Innovative Nutrition
1-866-526-7353 or (806) 355-5380
P.O. Box 21103, Amarillo, TX 79114

Adenosonine Monophosphate Sublingual Tabs (AMP)		90 tabs	$39.95
Lipotropic		100 count	$29.95
Calcium pyruvate	500mg	200 count	$24.99
Chitosan	500mg	120 count	$22.50
Carniforskolin		60 count	$44.95
Master Fiber & Herbal Blend		12 oz.	$19.95
Green Tea	315mg	100 count	$15.95
Omega-3 Fatty Acid	1000mg	100 count	$24.95
Bio-Citrin	500mg	90 count	$34.95
Hoodia gordonii		60 count	$39.95

Conjugated Linoleic Acid (CLA)	1000mg	120 count	$42.95
Gamma Linolenoic Acid	300mg	180 count	$49.95
Prevenzyme		100 count	$29.95
Flaxseed Oil		8 oz.	$11.95

Mesunique and *Accelerator* can be purchased from Nuvo Concepts at www.nuvoconcepts.com and www.mesunique.com.

Physicians can obtain *MesoDerm* from Legere Pharmaceuticals, 1-800-528-3144.

About the Author

Dr. Parker is one of the preeminent physicians in the United States in the field of Mesotherapy. His training includes personally working under Dr. Jacque LeCoz of Paris, France, the foremost Mesotherapy authority in the world. In addition to training with Dr. LeCoz, Dr. Parker has trained with experts from Brazil, Venezuela, Canada and the United States. Dr. Parker is president of the North American Society of Meso-Lipotherapy, president of the North American College of Meso-Lipotherapy, and a member of the American Society of Aesthetic Mesotherapy.

Dr. Parker's background is wide-ranged. His specialties include preventive medicine, nutrition and weight loss, as well as hyperbaric oxygen and pain management. He was named 2003 Physician of the Year by the National Republican Congressional Committee's Physician Advisory Board.

He writes a health and wellness newsletter and has appeared on numerous television and radio programs such as *That's Incredible, The Today Show,* and *Ounce of Prevention.* Dr. Parker is listed in *Who's Who in the World* and *Who's Who in Medicine.*

Dr. Parker regularly trains physicians in his office in Mesotherapy and other techniques, and conducts training seminars for physicians from all over the United States.

He is co-developer of the TP109 Hyperbaric Oxygen Chamber.

He is a strong Christian and serves on the Board of Bible Heritage Christian School. He has a loving wife and four children. Three of his children are in the medical profession and his fourth child is a Baptist minister. He has ten wonderful grandchildren.

Dr. Parker can be reached at the following address:

The Doctor's Clinic
4714 S. Western
Amarillo, Texas 79109
(806) 355-8263

Or his Web site...
www.doctorsclinicamarillo.com